Fitness
After
Fifty

Fitness After Fifty

by

Elaine LaLanne

with Richard Benyo

THE STEPHEN GREENE PRESS
Lexington, Massachusetts

ACKNOWLEDGMENTS:

Richard and David for their assistance
in developing this concept;
my sons, Dan and Jon Allen,
and my daughter, Yvonne,
and my support crew: Katherine Bentley,
Liz Cardenas, Alma Ebbert, Hattie Montez,
Kevin Kerslake, and Risa Sheppard.

First published in 1986 by
The Stephen Greene Press, Inc.
Published simultaneously in Canada by
Penguin Books Canada Limited
Distributed by Viking Penguin Inc.,
40 West 23rd Street, New York, NY 10010

Printed in the United States of America by
The Murray Printing Co., Westford,
Massachusetts
Set in Palatino

DEDICATION:

To my husband,
Jack,
whose inspiration
(and perspiration)
has kept me youthful
and enabled me
to reach the highest
levels of spiritual,
emotional and
physical being.

Elaine LaLanne

One of the most difficult jobs in the world is keeping up with Elaine LaLanne. She is one of the most well-known proponents of the fitness lifestyle, who practices what she preaches. Even though constantly on the move, she has for the last 30-plus years fully participated in raising three children, as well as running two households. She makes personal appearances, lectures, and accompanies her husband throughout the country, besides having co-hosted the nationally syndicated *Jack LaLanne Show.* Elaine runs several businesses based on health and fitness, still leaving time for her favorite charities.

Elaine began her career as a radio actress in 1946. Two years later she began working as a model and as record coordinator for the then fledgling 45 rpm division at RCA Victor. She moved into television in 1950 as co-host of a 90-minute daily variety show on the ABC affiliate in San Francisco; the show was the forerunner of the popular talk and variety shows of today.

Three years later, she became an executive at KVSM radio in San Mateo, California, conducting her own radio show and selling radio time. While doing the TV variety show, she'd met Jack LaLanne, whom she credits with changing her life. "I thought I was pretty fit," she says, recalling those days. "But Jack showed me that my diet was a mess and that my body proportions could be improved by a regular exercise program. Once I got my proportions built to where they should be, I began working to keep them there." By keeping a regular fitness program, Elaine has managed to maintain those proportions for more than 25 years.

It is her feeling that fitness must be made a regular part of your everyday life that prompted her to put together her *Fitness After Fifty* as an aid to the millions of fitness proponents across the country.

Despite their hectic lecturing, personal appearances and work schedule, the LaLannes manage to carve out a portion of time each week that they can spend quietly together, enjoying each other's company away from the rest of the world.

Contents

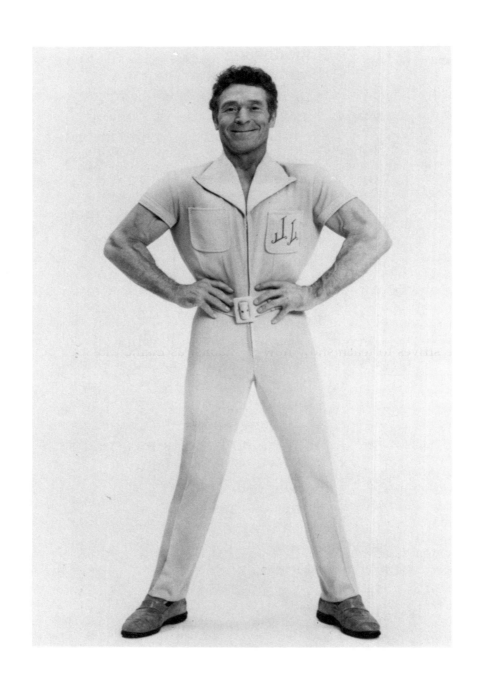

Foreword

Perhaps I'm a little prejudiced, but to my way of thinking, my wife Elaine is a tremendous example of what fitness is all about. If you are around her for any length of time, you will find that her enthusiasm for life is a very contagious thing—and it's all due to fitness!

She is very seldom down or depressed; her enthusiasm for life is wonderful. She has control of her mind, body, and spirit, and is totally dedicated to physical fitness and nutrition. In all these things, she is holistically sound. Not only is Elaine sound intellectually, she is a very social person, with a great personality—she sincerely loves people and they love her. To me, she is the living proof of all that a woman can be. Physically, she can do fifty push-ups and makes chin-ups look easy; she's a terrific golfer, an expert water skier and swimmer, a super wife and a good friend. She is a lecturer, author, civic leader, and an expert businessperson. She personifies the two qualities in life that combine so she cannot fail: pride and discipline!

In her book, she strives to teach/show how to attain these attributes. Once pride and discipline have been developed, the path that lies ahead will be easier and you will be a success at anything you undertake. In Elaine's program you'll learn to grow. I don't mean in girth; rather, to grow like the trees and plants grow. If we nourish the trees and the plants and obey nature's laws, they will flourish. So it is with the human body; if we obey nature's laws and nourish our bodies properly, with exercise and nutrition, our bodies will also grow to be more beautiful and healthy.

This program is three books in one. It is a personal diary, a recipe book, and an exercise book.

It is a diary you can begin any time of the year. You don't have to wait until January. You are not working alone; you and Elaine are working together. She not only gives you inspiration, but exercises which reach all the muscle groups. She shares with you her secrets on preparing easy recipes, which generally take less than a half-hour. In fact, she offers you a celebration feast every three months. No matter what your present level of fitness is, there is something here for everyone.

When I first met Elaine over thirty years ago, she was working on *The Les Malloy Show*, a ninety-minute afternoon television show in San Francisco. She was not only programming the show, but also appearing on it as well. She was smoking cigarettes and eating junk food. One day she decided to change all that. She stopped smoking, changed her eating habits and started on a regular exercise routine. Within the first month, she saw visible signs of reshaping her body. She did a total reversal. Her complete dedication to her profession stems from seeing her youth slipping away at a young age of 27. You, too, can reverse your lifestyle and eating habits, as Elaine did, and develop a positive, new image. This can all be achieved by following her lead in *Fitness After Fifty*.

Jack LaLanne

Introduction

People in developed nations are living longer than ever these days. In many nations, people are living twice as long as they did at the beginning of this century. Medical science has worked wonders eliminating the common and widespread diseases that had for years killed people in their prime. Now that the years a person can expect to live has increased significantly, it is time to bring quality into those precious, extra years. It is high time we disproved the myth that life after 50 is a life on the physical and mental decline, and that at 60 you can—and should—be put out to pasture (a pleasant euphemism for ignored).

Fortunately, we are living in the golden age of enlightenment when it comes to health and fitness. The same medical/scientific community that found cures for many fatal diseases is currently turning out reams of information on the benefits of a fit, healthy lifestyle. The spotlight of enlightenment has shown that there is an incredible potential for physical improvement beyond one's 50th birthday. In some ways, the mature person who is fit is able to make a lie of the old saying that "youth is wasted on the young," because if you feel young, you can live a youthful life. To quote my husband, "Some people die at 30 and they bury them at 90."

The over-50 person, armed with my basic fitness program of regular exercise, good nutrition, and a positive outlook toward life, can quite literally recapture the vigor of youth, turning the second half of life into the best years of life.

This book is the response to the increasing frequency of this question: "Elaine, I'm in my 50s. Is it too late for me to get fit and stay fit?"

The answer is a resounding, "No, it's not too late!"

I like to think that we have three ages:

1. Chronological age: Actual age in years
2. Physical age: How you feel at present
3. Psychological age: How you feel mentally

I personally stick with the physical because when I feel physically young, it helps me feel psychologically young. I seldom think about my chronological age. I try to think of the year in my life when I felt the greatest . . . then I set my mind to that feeling, picture it and strive for it. That age in my life was 19. I was talking to a couple of friends the other day; they are in their 60s, and they feel the same way I do about age. He thought of himself as 24, his wife 21. Why not picture your greatest year and strive for that feeling?

In the early 1940s I was swimming in the Minneapolis Aqua Follies and was in good condition. But by the time I first met Jack in the early 1950s at the age of 27, I thought I was old . . . over the hill. I was working at the ABC-TV station in San Francisco as a Girl Friday on the Les Malloy Show. The show was on from 4:30 to 6:30 p.m. every day and I not only booked the show but also appeared on it. At that time, I was the full support of my two children, so the strain of running a household and holding down a job didn't leave much time for caring about my eating or exercising habits. Consequently, I was a junk food junkie . . . living on Danish rolls and chocolate doughnuts for breakfast. For lunch: candy bars and soft drinks from the vending machines. For dinner: a hot dog or maybe a can of roast beef, a can of vegetables and ice cream. I was not eating any fresh vegetables or fresh fruit, and my skin was beginning to show it. I thought when you age, you just age, and nothing can be done about it.

Jack joined the TV gang at KGO-TV about a year after I did. Our mutual office was in the newsroom. Each day, Jack would come in filled with enthusiasm, talking with his director about his life-long profession, while I was down at the other end of the room smoking my cigarettes, eating my chocolate doughnut and worrying about who I was going to get to replace a last-minute cancellation. I heard LaLanneisms like: "Ten seconds on the lips and a lifetime on the hips" . . . "Use or lose" . . . "Wear nature's girdle" . . . "The food you eat today is walking and talking tomorrow" . . . "Your waistline is your lifeline." One day while I was indulging, he said to me: "You should be eating apples and bananas and oranges. If I didn't like you, I wouldn't tell you this."

I looked up at him while puffing on my cigarette and said: "Oh yeah!"

After that, I started thinking about my life, and the way I looked (my chestline was sinking into my waistline, while my legs were getting that washboard look). I really felt old. Suddenly, I wanted to be 19 again; maybe something really could be done! I went home that night and took off all my clothes and stood in front of a mirror and realized the awful truth about myself and decided that *something had to be done*!

Well, the end of this little story is that I started exercising every day at a class Jack conducted at noontime for a few interested people at the studio. I quit smoking, broiled everything I used to fry, cut out all white sugar and white flour products. In one month I saw the changes that had taken place in my body.

My skin became smoother and tighter. I reproportioned my body through exercise and diet. My eyesight even became more acute: blues were bluer, greens were greener. I'm sure this had to do with my quitting smoking; as I understand it, smoking constricts the blood vessels in your eyes. Suddenly, I was a convert! I, too, wanted to preach this message to all who would listen. You see, I started slowing the aging process way back then. I'd hate to think of what I would look like today if I hadn't met Jack. His LaLanneisms, "You eat every day, you sleep every day, your body was made to exercise every day," have stuck with me all these years. I now eat every day, sleep every day, and *exercise* every day.

There is evidence all around us of people from 40 to 80 years of age, even into their 90s, who literally bubble over with enthusiasm, energy and health, and a zest for life that would startle the average 20-year-old.

Yes, you'll say, but these are special people. They were born with genes that make them biologically superior to me. That may or may not be true. Jack LaLanne was not always the Jack LaLanne everyone knows; at one time, Jack was your typical 98-pound weakling, but he decided to do something about it.

Even if you have the best genes in the world, they will take you only so far. The older you become, the more it becomes a matter of consistently working at being at your best, both physically and mentally.

The wonderful thing about the human body is its willingness to adapt. If you demand nothing of it, it will be very satisfied to adapt to nothing. It's the realization of the theory, "Use it or lose it." Too many people allow themselves to lose it and then blame the loss on everything else they can think of. If you don't use the heart muscle, pretty soon you're going to find it losing its ability to function well. On the other hand, if you do use it, you'll find it adapting to the demands you're placing on it.

This book is designed especially for the person over 50 who is in relatively stable health, and who wants to use his or her body effectively and well.

The human body isn't built with its largest, most powerful muscles in the legs just so it can sit around all day on its behind. The large muscles in the legs are there because the human body was made to move!, to be kinetic!, to be dynamic!, to be alive! You'll have plenty of time to lie around like deadwood after you die. In the meantime, live! And in living, train yourself to live life and enjoy life as a healthy, fit human being.

Go to your family doctor for a thorough physical examination and seek his advice on the pace at which it is safe for you to begin a fitness program.

It is never too late to start; and by starting, you gain some very positive results.

Elaine LaLanne
Hollywood, California
March 1986

Defining "fitness"

Defining "fitness" is sort of like defining "love." It is almost impossible to come up with a definition that applies to everyone. Fitness is many things to many people.

My definition of "fitness" is a combination of a lot of things, including proper exercise, diet, rest, attitude and spiritual and emotional peace. In other words, it's the maximum you! You need all these things to be that maximum! For instance, you're not the maximum if you lose weight and don't exercise. As a result, you become weak, flabby and soft. Remember, exercise gives the body energy.

My husband, Jack, puts it this way: "Fitness is waking up in the morning with a song in your heart, a smile on your face, no aches or pains. You work all day and still have the energy to do the things your mind wants to, when you want to do it."

Fitness is a matter of being prepared. It is an insurance policy. It's the Fountain of Youth! If you are physically and mentally fit, you can almost reverse the aging process.

The state of fitness is unique to each of us, because each of us was born a unique creature with a unique body. Just as no two grains of sand are exactly alike, so no two bodies are exactly alike. Each body has its own unique potential. Everyone is capable of achieving some level of fitness—a fitness that is right and correct for that person alone.

In this program, that person is YOU! Because you are the only person who can truly be responsible for your fitness. You cannot depend on someone else to get you fit or keep you fit. You must cultivate a knowledge of fitness in order to understand what fitness is and what it can do for you and how it can change your life for the better.

But you must *want* fitness for your body and for your mind. You must *want* to reward your body for having been fortunate enough to be given into the custody of such a genuinely concerned person.

I get very excited when I talk about fitness to people like you—people who have made the commitment to get fit, to get truly alive, to take care of themselves!

There are too many people in life who like to spend all their time sliding along, only to come to the end of it, where they feel cheated because they didn't get as much out of it as they'd have liked. Well, that person probably didn't realize that we only go through this life once, that we're only given one body to make that trip, and that we'd better take care of it. And when we take care of it, it is marvelous how well it takes care of us, both physically and mentally.

A fit body helps us to feel better, it helps us to take more pride in ourselves and it makes many things possible that would have been totally impossible otherwise.

That's what I mean by defining "fitness" as being *the state of the maximum you.*

Fitness, then, is when everything about you is kept well-tuned so that you can be the best physical person possible. By being a better person physically, you can be a better person in almost every other way.

This book is one year's volume in the history of *your* fitness, *your* life.

We've designed it so that you can waltz right into it at any time of the year and you can start your fitness record when *you* want to—not when someone else tells you or when the calendar dictates. A year from now, when you're ready to close the last page of this volume and start your next volume, you can page back through your own story, and I have the feeling that it will be quite an inspiring story!

Combining diet and exercise

Diet plus Exercise equals Fitness. Diet and exercise are what fitness is all about. They go hand in hand. Everyone knows that going on a diet can sometimes help you lose weight. But what do you look like after the weight loss? You've lost your muscle tone, strength and energy. In order to maintain—and even add to—these three, along with the diet, one must exercise as well as give the proper nourishment to those muscles.

Let's analyze the word ''diet.'' What does that word mean to you? Is it what you eat everyday? Or does it mean ''hungry,'' ''calories,'' ''temporary,'' or ''regimented eating''? When I think of the word ''diet,'' the first thought that comes into my mind is ''temporary.'' Most people who go on a diet end up going off and on and off and on. Lose weight, gain weight, lose weight, gain weight. A vicious cycle, and what have you accomplished? Instead of using the word ''diet,'' let's use the expression ''a way of life.''

There are many kinds of dieters:

1. **The Picker, Taster or Snacker.** ''Oh, I hardly eat anything all day and yet gain weight.'' How many times have you said or heard this? Well, if you're taking in more calories than you're burning up, you are going to gain weight. The Picker picks all day and each pick has calories. I like to compare The Picker to the newspaper business; when I was a child, newspapers were two cents. The newspaper empire was built on pennies, and The Picker builds a big corporation (usually in front) before he or she realizes it.

2. **One Meal a Day.** I've found that many people who do not eat all day long overeat at the evening meal, not realizing that they have ingested more calories than if they had eaten three regular meals.

3. **The Hidden Calories Dieter.** This dieter has very good intentions! This person drinks coffee with no cream, but loads it with sugar, prepares a cottage cheese salad for lunch and tops it off with pie a la mode, broils a steak and stuffs the 75-calorie baked potato with butter and sour cream.

4. **The Over-Indulger.** This person is very careful about food selection and buys everything that is healthy; however, he consumes too much at a sitting. For instance, as my husband Jack says, ''One apple a day is good, but why eat 100 of them?''

I have included some easy-to-fix recipes in this book. Eating good food doesn't necessarily mean you have to be in the kitchen all day. Although our family primarily eats chicken, fish or turkey, I occasionally eat meat, such as lamb stew, leg of lamb, and at times a lean beef patty.

On each week of this *Diary*, you'll find a recipe that I've gathered from years of experimenting. On pages 134-141, you'll find meals put together from these weekly recipes. These four sets of meals are what I like to think of as the seasonal victory meals. The diet and exercise program you are following should periodically be re-evaluated and new goals set. (We'll talk about goals on page xxiv.) I feel that four times a year is sufficient for re-evaluating and re-setting major goals. And what better time to do that than the first day of each new season of the year?

On the first day of Spring, I suggest you plan a meal as outlined on pages 134-135. Invite some of your friends over and have a meal in good cheer. Discuss with them your progress in your fitness program. Talk about setting reasonable goals for the spring season—goals that will be reflected in the notations in your *Diary*. As you're using your *Diary* to put together this meal, also use the *Diary* as a reference point for your discussions of where your fitness program has come over the last three months. Jot down these goals...

Proper diet is an integral part of your fitness program. Your body is very much like a machine. You can tune it perfectly, but if it isn't getting the correct fuel, it isn't going to run at its maximum. I like to ''earn my breakfast'' by putting off eating until I've done my exercises.

I urge you to try the recipes and exercises I've included in this *Diary*. By exercising and working some of these recipes into your daily routine, you can begin to weed out some of the undisciplined areas. *Bon appetit!*

Nutrition and the fit person

The word "diet" leaves a bad taste in the mouth. But ironically, the word "diet" does not technically refer to systematically depriving oneself of certain foods in an attempt to lose weight. The word "diet" refers, quite simply, to what we eat. A person with three percent body fat has a diet just as surely as people who weigh 300 pounds and stuff themselves with chocolate candies all day long.

It is only through obsession with weight loss that the word has been forced and twisted into a meaning that is associated with sacrifice and suffering and depriving oneself. Many dictionaries have even bowed to this popular meaning of the word.

For many Americans dieting has become a hobby, an avocation, an obsession. They try out new diets like they try on fashions for the new season. It seems that no one diet works for everyone! And for some people, no diet works at all. New books with the latest get-thin-quick diets fill the bestseller lists, with others waiting in the wings to get on the bandwagon when one that's listed weakens and slips. And so it goes...

Everytime I hear people say, "I'm on a diet," I immediately shudder and think, "Uh-oh...temporary...that can't last for the rest of their lives." I've seen too many people who are on the yo-yo bandwagon; they lose some, gain some, lose some, gain some... never really getting the results they desire, because they haven't changed their *way of life*. Try saying out loud to yourself, "I'm on a diet" and then, "I'm on a Way of Life." Which phrase would you be more apt to abide by?

Our bodies are truly remarkable. They have the ability to replace themselves every 90 days, so it stands to reason that what you put in your mouth today will show itself later. In an attempt to help the body, many people who diet actually weaken it by restricting the nutrients going into it. It's like planting a garden. "What you sow, so shall you reap." In order to perform its necessary functions, to produce energy, and to fight off sickness and disease, the body needs certain minimum nutrients every day. Getting those nutrients constitutes *good nutrition*.

We are all looking for an easy way. But what works for one does not work for another. I have found that the most important part of going on a diet, or a good nutritional program, or a way of life, is that the individual must make a personal commitment. That means if you think of "diet" as a temporary thing, your commitment is short-lived.

On the other hand, maybe you do want something that is temporary: a quick weight-loss diet that provides you with immediate results. It makes you feel better psychologically. By all means try it, but only if it is nutritionally sound. Stick with your commitment and taper off into a lifestyle when you have reached your goal.

Calories! What Are They? A calorie represents a specific amount of energy producing heat as a byproduct created by your body burning a specific amount of food. Which means, if you consume more calories a day than you burn, the excess calories will become stored fat.

Everyone should be familiar with a calories chart. You don't necessarily have to know the calorie count of each portion of food you ingest, but the fact that it is either high or low in calories. Try to develop an appetite for the lower calorie foods, keeping the high calorie foods to a minimum.

An easy way to start out is to put foods in groups such as vegetables, fruits, whole grains, dairy products, meats, poultry and fish. In each category, learn to know whether the count is high or low. Each time you start to take a bit of a high calorie food, say to yourself, "What is this doing for me? Will it make me slim and trim or will it just add more pounds to my body?" This is something I have made part of my life. I always ask myself, "What is this food going to do for me?" Or, "Is it sound nutritionally?".

Although I do not count calories per se, I *do*

know that calories count...just like 2 plus 2 equals 4; they can add up...and up...and up.

Not only do calories count, so do the kinds of calories you ingest. You can lose weight on 1000 calories a day of either candy bars or nutritional foods. However, from the candy bars you will suffer hunger pangs much more than if you were eating more nutritiously. Your body is telling you it needs much more than just empty calories. Also, those empty calories can bring about mood swings or personality changes. Your blood sugar goes up and stays up for a short while, then drops way down—you get that sinking feeling. On the other hand, if you ingest low calorie but nutritious foods, your blood sugar goes up and stays there even for a matter of hours. Good nutrition gives you more food value for your calories—so more value for your money, also.

What Is Blood Sugar? Simply defined in the dictionary and without getting too technical, blood sugar is the glucose or dextrose in the blood that rises and falls depending upon what you eat. All food must be converted to be used by the body. The glucose or sugar level in the blood is what is readily available for energy for the brain and muscles. Ideally, we would like to have an even, high level of energy all day long to enjoy work and play to the best of our abilities. This is achieved by eating slowly digested complex carbohydrates, fats and proteins. Refined sugar raises the blood level rapidly and dramatically, but due to its high concentration it overloads the system and soon causes a rapid fall to below normal. This can cause irritability, depression, grouchiness, or just plain fatigue. I can remember having these feelings when I was eating sweets and junk foods.

No diet or program of good nutrition works effectively unless it is coupled with a program of exercise. Daily exercise routines will help to increase your rate of burning extra fat calories that your body has stored. For example, swimming can burn up to 400 or 675 calories per hour, running can burn up to 650 to 900 calories per hour, cycling 420 calories per hour and a fast walk, 330 calories per hour. Watching television, on the other hand, burns only 40 calories per hour. So, it looks like the handwriting is on the wall. You need a program of exercise to help burn excess calories.

Is Age A Factor? Yes, the older you get the fewer calories your body requires. This usually happens both because your metabolism slows with age and your physical activities are not as vigorous as when you were younger. More handwriting on the wall...you *need* a program of exercise.

We need exercise for other reasons as well; it helps us to better assimilate our food and get more nutrition for fewer calories and less money. It also helps normalize appetite, promote regularity, metabolize and utilize vitamins and minerals, along with helping us to sleep better. Exercise also fights degenerative diseases (aging), arteriosclerosis (hardening of the arteries) and high blood pressure. To sum it all up, exercise and nutrition go hand in hand.

About The Recipes. The recipes in this book are not necessarily designed to be low calorie diet dishes, but to be simple and easy to fix, while still being very nutritious. There are so many myths about nutritious foods, such as potatoes...It seems that all my life I've heard that potatoes are fattening. It's not the potato that is fattening, but what you put on the potato. A medium sized potato is 75–100 calories; a banana is only about 100 calories. We also use some foods that are higher in calories but exceptionally nutritious, such as the avocado. One avocado is approximately 425 calories, but how many people eat the whole avocado? Most avocado recipes call for slices. Avocados are exceptionally high in vitamins and minerals, as is non-refined brown rice. One cup of brown rice has about the same calories as half an avocado, is lower in calories than white rice, and is loaded with nutritional food value.

Regularity and commitment to a program

Look in any dictionary. The majority of definitions for commitment boil down to one thing: performance. How has your commitment translated into performance? Whether you are overweight or underweight, your goals are ultimately defined by your performance record. Whatever your commitment, it is the end result of this record of performance that you must live with. Therefore, if you make a commitment to good health and then turn it around by saying, "Well, I have no will power," and every day you say to yourself, "I'll start my program tomorrow," you are defeated before you start. Remember, that *we all have will power!* You willed yourself to get out of bed this morning, to brush your teeth, to get dressed. Each thing we do during the day takes will power. Just reach out to yourself and use your powers to reshape yourself.

Make a commitment. Teach yourself to enjoy it. My father always used to tell me that "someone who enjoys what he or she does will do it well."

This especially applies to something like fitness. If you learn to like it, you'll do it well, and it will become an extremely important part of your life. I don't personally love working out, but every time I do it I think of the results and it's easier. Think of the results and work toward goals.

Let's face it, it isn't very much fun getting started. But again, think of the results. It takes a very special person to be able to take charge of his or her life, and you're one of those special people. Keep that in mind. When you begin your exercise program, remember that you're working against the scientific principle that a body at rest tends to stay at rest. This is called "inertia." You've got to overcome this.

There is another scientific principle that you can bring into play, however: a body in motion tends to stay in motion, until acted upon by some outside force. So the more you move, the more you get into your program, the easier it will be.

I started working out years ago with simple calisthenics and I saw results within two weeks. Once I moved up to using weights for my training, within a mere three months I had managed to completely reproportion my body.

So, if you're just starting your fitness program, please don't become discouraged if you do not become slim and supple the first week. Stick with it. Make it a way of life. Believe me, it's worth it, because it will rebuild your entire life from this day forward. You will take over control of your own life again. It's the best thing you'll ever do for yourself—the best present you can give yourself.

And one of the best ways I know to make fitness work for you and to fulfill that commitment is to get into a *regular* schedule of fitness from the start. In starting your exercise program, one good rule to follow is "crawl, walk, and then run." In other words, start out very easily and increase the intensity and repetition as your physical condition improves. I don't want you to get stiff and sore and overly tired at first. If you feel you can do an exercise 10 times, start out by cutting that number in half; then each succeeding day, strive to do more.

Regularity is very important because without it, your fitness isn't going to physically take hold. Fitness demands regularity for it to work. Keep track of your exercise work pattern in your diary. Make your commitment now and stick with it!

Music and exercise

I'm sure that you have heard the expression, "Music soothes the savage beast."

To my way of thinking, a world without music would be a world not worth experiencing. Music adds a whole 'nother dimension to life. Its diversity offers something for everyone, from the Boston Pops to rock 'n' roll, big band music to jazz, country & Western to the classics.

What's fascinating about music is that it gets your feet moving, no matter what type of music it is. I've seen people in elegant evening clothes at a concert hall tapping their toes to classical music with just as much feeling as the younger generation responds to the latest top 40 hit.

My first job during high school was folding papers for the Sears-Roebuck advertiser. Now folding papers sounds like a pretty boring thing to do, except for the fact that the company played the latest music in the background. I found it was possible to make a game out of it. Folding papers to the beat of the music was fun. In fact, I looked forward to coming to work. (Sears was one of the pioneers in playing music for their employees...) There are negatives in everything we do, but on the other hand, there are also positives. Too many people dwell on the negatives and forget about the positives. In my case, music was certainly a positive, and it did much to wipe out the negative: boredom. I try to always dwell on the positive, and it certainly makes life much happier.

Today, music continues to soothe office workers and patrons in banks and other such public buildings. In institutions, music is found to work in calming patients. We all know it's terrific for a long drive in the automobile and it certainly has a very special place in churches.

It also meshes beautifully with exercising and fitness. Music is the backbone of Jazzercise and Aerobic Dance and all other similar exercise classes.

Jack and I have always used music while exercising at home or on our television show; it makes a wonderful backdrop for doing exercises. So why not match your music to your mood when you exercise at home? You need days when your exercises are done slowly and easily, more to keep you loose than to really build strength. Those are the days when your muscles may be a little sore from particularly ambitious workouts the day before and need some tender loving care to recuperate. On those days, it's nice to put some slow, easy music on the stereo, and do your exercises at the same slow, easy pace, working toward flexibility, saving the vigorous exercise for the next day.

Then, there are days, of course, when you're really up and you really want to exercise. Put on something lively and let it rip!

It's also nice every once in a while to invite friends over to do a half-hour of exercises with you.

Perhaps you are one of those people who likes to come up with specific routines of specific lengths and specific tempos. If you have a tape machine, make tapes of your music rather than having to go through a batch of record albums.

What a wonderful feeling to put on a good tape and to let yourself really get carried away by creating your own exercise routine. Flow with the music, go with its movements, let it carry you through your routine.

When a certain routine really moves you, you'll want to make note of it in your *Diary* so that you can go back to it occasionally and attempt to re-create the sensation and the success of that routine.

Also, be sure to experiment. You might find that you can develop a liking for a certain type of music you never cared for before. Strike up the band, and let's get fit!

This week covers _____ , _____ , _____ , to _____ , _____ , _____ .
month   day   year   month   day   year

Monday	E X E R C I S E	Activity _____ _____ Time _____ Distance _____ Pace _____ Effort: ☐ Easy ☐ Moderate ☐ Hard ☐ Extreme	Remarks (fitness): _____ _____ _____ Remarks (personal): _____ _____ _____
Resting Pulse Rate / Weight At Rising			

Tuesday	E X E R C I S E	Activity _____ _____ Time _____ Distance _____ Pace _____ Effort: ☐ Easy ☐ Moderate ☐ Hard ☐ Extreme	Remarks (fitness): _____ _____ _____ Remarks (personal): _____ _____ _____
Resting Pulse Rate / Weight At Rising			

Wednesday	E X E R C I S E	Activity _____ _____ Time _____ Distance _____ Pace _____ Effort: ☐ Easy ☐ Moderate ☐ Hard ☐ Extreme	Remarks (fitness): _____ _____ _____ Remarks (personal): _____ _____ _____
Resting Pulse Rate / Weight At Rising			

Thursday	E X E R C I S E	Activity _____ _____ Time _____ Distance _____ Pace _____ Effort: ☐ Easy ☐ Moderate ☐ Hard ☐ Extreme	Remarks (fitness): _____ _____ _____ Remarks (personal): _____ _____ _____
Resting Pulse Rate / Weight At Rising			

Friday	E X E R C I S E	Activity _____ _____ Time _____ Distance _____ Pace _____ Effort: ☐ Easy ☐ Moderate ☐ Hard ☐ Extreme	Remarks (fitness): _____ _____ _____ Remarks (personal): _____ _____ _____
Resting Pulse Rate / Weight At Rising			

Saturday	E X E R C I S E	Activity _____ _____ Time _____ Distance _____ Pace _____ Effort: ☐ Easy ☐ Moderate ☐ Hard ☐ Extreme	Remarks (fitness): _____ _____ _____ Remarks (personal): _____ _____ _____
Resting Pulse Rate / Weight At Rising			

Sunday	E X E R C I S E	Activity _____ _____ Time _____ Distance _____ Pace _____ Effort: ☐ Easy ☐ Moderate ☐ Hard ☐ Extreme	Remarks (fitness): _____ _____ _____ Remarks (personal): _____ _____ _____
Resting Pulse Rate / Weight At Rising			

Sample Diary page

This week covers _Jan._, _16_, _1984_, to _Jan._, _22_, _1984_.
(month) (day) (year) (month) (day) (year)

Monday	E X E R C I S E	**Activity** Gym / Pool exercises **Time** Gym 20 min. / Pool 15 min. **Distance** ____ **Pace** Fast / moderate **Effort:** ☒ Easy ☐ Moderate ☐ Hard ☐ Extreme	**Remarks (fitness):** Pool 58° — only one lap. Brrr... Did pool exercises in hot tub. **Remarks (personal):** Remember to call brother tomorrow.
Resting Pulse Rate 72 / **Weight At Rising** 117			

Tuesday	E X E R C I S E	**Activity** Calisthenics / Golf **Time** 15 min. / 3 hours **Distance** — / 6,000 yds. **Pace** Fast / Fast **Effort:** ☐ Easy ☒ Moderate ☐ Hard ☐ Extreme	**Remarks (fitness):** Went around course in 3 hours (walking). My 15 min. workout seemed to give me more energy. **Remarks (personal):** Feel like celebrating. Shot 87. Have been in slump lately.
Resting Pulse Rate 70 / **Weight At Rising** 116			

Wednesday	E X E R C I S E	**Activity** Gym / hot tub / pool exercise **Time** 20 min. **Distance** ____ **Pace** slow / Fast **Effort:** ☐ Easy ☐ Moderate ☒ Hard ☐ Extreme	**Remarks (fitness):** Changed program in gym. Working harder on backs of thighs. **Remarks (personal):** Benefit committee meeting — 30 people for light supper at house. 7-11 pm. To bed at 1am. Too late!
Resting Pulse Rate 72 / **Weight At Rising** 118			

Thursday	E X E R C I S E	**Activity** Stretching + Gym **Time** 30 min. **Distance** ____ **Pace** ____ **Effort:** ☐ Easy ☐ Moderate ☒ Hard ☐ Extreme	**Remarks (fitness):** Sore from new workout. Hard to get through it. Tired from last night. **Remarks (personal):** Proud of myself for sticking with the workout. Felt like a million afterwards.
Resting Pulse Rate 84* / **Weight At Rising** 118			

Friday	E X E R C I S E	**Activity** Jogging — running — fast walking **Time** 25 min. **Distance** 2 miles **Pace** Slow-fast-slow-fast **Effort:** ☐ Easy ☐ Moderate ☒ Hard ☐ Extreme	**Remarks (fitness):** Back of legs still sore from Wednesday workout. Did some extra stretching. **Remarks (personal):** Felt sad today. Heard that M.G. was in bad car accident. Thought about Janet.
Resting Pulse Rate 74 / **Weight At Rising** 117			

Saturday	E X E R C I S E	**Activity** Aerobics to / Eve. music / dancing **Time** 45 min. / 1 hour **Distance** ____ **Pace** moderate / Fast **Effort:** ☒ Easy ☐ Moderate ☐ Hard ☐ Extreme	**Remarks (fitness):** Planning aerobics routines for May cruise. **Remarks (personal):** Had a great time dancing tonight. Hadn't been dancing in ages.
Resting Pulse Rate 72 / **Weight At Rising** 117			

Sunday	E X E R C I S E	**Activity** Bicycling **Time** 30 min. **Distance** 4 miles **Pace** Moderate **Effort:** ☐ Easy ☐ Moderate ☒ Hard ☐ Extreme	**Remarks (fitness):** Had not been bicycling in a couple of months due to holidays. Felt great. **Remarks (personal):** Went to Lucy's memorial service. I'll miss her very much.
Resting Pulse Rate 74 / **Weight At Rising** 116			

* Resting pulse rate up — probably due to late night the night before and change in workout program.

Goals and personal observations

The definition of a "goal" is "that toward which effort is directed." A personal observation, on the other hand, is "the art of noticing or perceiving something about yourself."

I've grouped these two topics together for a very simple reason. Both are incredibly important to any fitness program, and both must come from deep within you.

Goals are set from within—they are your ultimate aims or desires. Your observations are your personal perceptions of how well you are doing—or have done—in accomplishing these goals.

A fitness program without goals is like a boat without a rudder. When a boat has a rudder, the rudder can be used to aim the boat toward a goal on the horizon, and the boat will proceed toward that goal unerringly. Too many people are going 'round haphazardly, playing around in their boat without really knowing how or where to steer it, until their desire for a goal fashions a rudder that allows them to plot a good course.

In any fitness program, you must initially have the desire to look and feel better. It's also important to set a course toward that desire or goal and then follow through. See yourself as you want to be. See the end result in your mind's eye. Imagine it already accomplished so that the goal pictured is clear and sharp!

The end result is going to be whatever you want it to be. For instance, if you love and crave sweets, you already know the consequences.

Here's a tip I always give in my lectures: Before that sweet reaches your mouth, ask yourself, "What is this going to do for me?" Another tip to help you reach your goal is to tape your picture to the refrigerator door. Then, every time you open it for a snack, close it quickly, and say to yourself, "Hey, self, I'm trying not to look like that anymore. Gimme a break!"

Both Jack and I encourage two types of goals: long-range goals and short-range goals. And coupled with the goals must be a certain flexibility. If something comes up so that you can't meet your goals on schedule, don't get discouraged. Stand back, observe, regroup, forge ahead and readjust your goals. I'd encourage you to break your year down into workable segments. For instance, twelve 30-day periods, six 60-day periods, or four 90-day periods. It makes a full year more manageable.

Every three months, I have designed a seasonal victory menu for the day. That special day with its special meals is designed as a time to evaluate your progress and it allows you to set your goals for your next victory day meal.

You'll also notice that there are spaces for goals on each left-hand page of each week of the diary. That is space for your short-term goals.

Long-term goals can be as simple as wanting to lose one inch around your waist during a three-month period; short-term goals can be as simple as wanting to do three more sit-ups per exercise session by the end of a week.

Your personal observations could also be called "truth in living." When you look at yourself, be critical, yes, but don't go overboard to the point where you discourage yourself, either. When you look in the mirror in the morning, challenge yourself. Make the mirror your friend. Talk to it. Ask yourself: "Am I on the way to accomplishing my goal?" Don't make excuses. One excuse leads to another and nothing gets accomplished and again in the end the only person who gets shortchanged is you. So make all observations honestly and fairly and you'll thank yourself in the end.

In evaluating your goals, did you reach them for this week or not? If your goal for this week was to do three more sit-ups per session, and you *almost* did them, but it was more like 2¾ sit-ups, then simply reset your goal for the next week. Believe me, when you actually do those three sit-ups cleanly and honestly, you'll just about burst with pride.

Using your resting pulse rate

The body is truly a wonderful thing. The harder it works, the stronger it becomes. What other machine can say that?

The body's capacity for work is defined by the ability of the heart to supply nourishment to the working muscles and to take away waste material. Each time the heart pumps, oxygen and nutrients are pumped out through the arteries to all parts of the body, and once the blood gets there, it exchanges the oxygen and nutrients for waste products to take back toward the heart. The efficiency with which the heart pumps and does its job has a great deal to do with how well your entire body works—and how long it will work.

Besides being able to feel your heart beating by placing your hand over it, there are other points in the body where you can feel this vital pulse. The most common spot, of course, is the wrist. The radial artery in the wrist is easy to locate. Turn your hand palm up. Now, using two fingers from your opposite hand, feel for the bone on the thumb side of the wrist. Move your fingers to just inside this bone, and you've found the radial artery. Feel it pumping? (You don't want to feel for it using your thumb on your opposite hand, because your thumb is large enough that it has its own pulse and it will disrupt your being able to feel the pulse.) If you want to take your pulse, check the second hand on your watch, and count pulse beats for 10 seconds and then multiply by six. The average person has a resting (pulse taken while sitting or lying down) pulse rate of about 70.

If you are going to engage in an aerobic sport, such as running or cycling or swimming, and you want to stay within a safe range of exertion, your pulse rate can be a guide. You want to exert yourself 60-70% of your maximum pulse rate. Let's look at how you determine that.

Start with the number 220. Now, subtract your age from that number. Let's say you're 40 years old. So your number would be 180. That's your maximum pulse rate. Your base training pulse rate (60-70% of maximum) would then be 108-126 beats per minute.

According to Amby Burfoot, 1968 winner of the Boston Marathon, in an article in *Runner's World*, this is considered the "safety zone," where you are strengthening the heart and not overstressing it. To determine whether or not you are staying in this range during a workout, stop periodically and count your pulse for 10 seconds and multiply by six.

This is not the only thing your pulse rate can do, however. Besides being a very good guide for keeping you within that "safety zone," you can and should use it as an indicator of whether you are working yourself too hard. You do this by regularly taking your resting pulse rate first thing in the morning. You'll notice on your *Diary* pages that there is a place for your morning resting pulse rate. This can be very important and very helpful to you.

Keep your watch by your bedside. As soon as you wake up, reach for your watch, lie back in your bed and allow yourself a minute or so to recover from the shock of waking up. Then take your pulse for a full 60 seconds. Your heart should be beating with a steady rhythm because nothing has happened yet in your day to throw it off.

So what is significant about taking your morning pulse rate?

After you have taken it, every day for one week, you will begin to see your pattern. If it is within a few beats, one way or another, you can figure that this reflects your resting pulse rate. But what happens if you wake up one morning and it is up ten points or more? It is an indication that your body may be making repairs, for some reason, and you should not plan on a strenuous workout that day. Back off and do an easier workout until your pulse rate comes back down within five points of your normal rate. Work toward the goal of lowering your pulse rate, in the course of six months or one year. It will be a sign that your regular exercising is making your heart and the rest of your body more efficient.

Fitness at 50 and beyond
Exercise Level 1

The one unchanging rule about a fitness program—any fitness program—is that it must constantly be changed in order to work. It must evolve with the person who is following it so that it can accommodate that person's progress—and that person's backsliding. There are more than 600 muscles in the body and each one needs its ration of work in order to keep it strong and healthy. If you do the same exercises constantly, the muscles you are working get used to working in exactly the same way and develop a narrow range of motion, while those that are not used become weak and almost useless. By constantly updating your program to your progress, muscles will be challenged in a different way and they will respond more readily.

This is especially true for people over 50 years of age who are exercising regularly. And that is why I've designed a three-level exercise program, featuring four weeks of exercise per level. Each program level features 12 specific exercises, which I call the Daily Dozen.

You will notice that each level also features extra pages so you can design your own program for those stubborn areas which need work. Simply fill in exercises from the Daily Dozen that work problem areas, or look up other exercises later in the book that would help bring problem areas into line. Or, you may know some exercises of your own that would work. Fill them in on the appropriate blank lines. For instance, if you have trouble with flabby thighs, fill in one or two thigh exercises under the Thigh category; examples would be Leg Lunges on page 26 or Half Squats on page 28. Then, you can use this specific body area program in conjunction with the daily program I've outlined, or you can use it separately.

Or, the blank pages can be used to create a Level 4 (and beyond) that concentrates on areas you feel need more work. This allows you to design programs specifically geared to your own needs and goals. (Don't hesitate to use a copying machine to copy these exercise pages so you can slip them into the week you're on in the diary section of this book; that saves you paging back and forth, and allows you to reuse the Exercise Program pages by simply copying more of them as needed.)

And finally, if you find the repetitions given too easy or too difficult, add more reps on the easy ones and cut down repetitions on the more difficult ones.

This program is designed as a guide for people 50 or older who have a minimum of exercise experience. It is advised, however, that before beginning the program, you consult a physician in order to determine your current capabilities for exercise. Then begin the week's schedule at a gentle pace that allows you to remain comfortable. In other words, make haste slowly. The complete program should take about six or seven minutes a day—certainly a modest investment in your health and fitness.

At the end of the first week, if you do not yet feel ready to move on to week two, don't feel you are being forced to do so. Stay at week one until you feel ready to progress. As a guide to your readiness to move on, monitor your pulse rate (p. xxv) and assess how you feel.

You'll find a page reference with each exercise that guides you to a detailed explanation—and a photo or two—of how to properly do the exercise. Feel free to frequently check your form, and recheck how to do the exercises. And don't get discouraged. Remember that in the beginning, you must mix one dose of determination with two doses of patience; patience wins the race.

Week 1 and 2

Area Affected	Daily Dozen	Exercise and Description	Page Ref.	Week 1 Repetitions	Week 2 Repetitions
Overall Warm-Up	1	**Dynamic Swings:** Swing down through legs and up again.	2	5	10
Neck Chin	2	**Neck & Chin Firmer:** Put chin on chest while resisting with fingers on forehead.	4	5	10
Shoulders Neck	3	**Shoulder Shrugs:** Bring shoulders up to ears, hold, and relax.	6	10	15
Shoulders Arms Neck Chest	4	**Arm Circles, Arm Crosses & Hand Extensions:** Extend arms, make circles, tense arms and cross in front; open and close hands.	8 12 16	10 each	15 each
Arms	5	**Back Arm Extensions:** Extend arms to the back, bend over at waist, elbows high, and extend arms toward ceiling.	14	4	8
Waist	6	**Side Bends:** Bend from waist to the left and then to the right.	18	10 ea. side	15 ea. side
Warm-Up Waist Thighs Legs	7	**Running in Place:** Stand tall and run in place, lifting legs high. If you cannot jog or run, march in place. Easy does it.	34	20 sec.	30 sec.
Hips Thighs	8	**Half Squats:** Hold on to a chair; bend knees, pause, straighten to standing position.	28	5	10
Legs	9	**Toe Raises:** Raise up on toes, hold for one count, and lower to original position.	32	10	15
Shoulders Arms Waist	10	**The Swimmer:** Bend over at waist, bend knees, bring arm up to ear, and pretend you are swimming.	64	20 sec.	30 sec.
Waist Arms Back	11	**Cobra Stretch:** Lie on floor or bed, then lift upper body with your arms; arch back, head up.	98	3	6
Warm-Down	12	**Rag Doll Relaxer:** Bend at waist while keeping back flat; arms hang loosely toward floor.	62	5 sec.	10 sec.

Week 3 and 4

Area Affected	Daily Dozen	Exercise and Description	Page Ref.	Week 3 Repetitions	Week 4 Repetitions
Overall Warm-Up	1	**Dynamic Swings:** Swing down through legs and up again.	2	15	20
Neck Chin	2	**Neck & Chin Firmer:** Put chin on chest while resisting with fingers on forehead.	4	15	20
Shoulders Neck	3	**Shoulder Shrugs:** Bring shoulders up to ears, hold, and relax.	6	20	25
Shoulders Arms Neck Chest	4	**Arm Circles, Arm Crosses & Hand Extensions:** Extend arms, make circles, tense arms and cross in front; open and close hands.	8 12 16	20 each	25 each
Arms	5	**Back Arm Extensions:** Extend arms to the back, bend over at waist, elbows high, and extend arms toward ceiling.	14	15	20
Waist	6	**Side Bends:** Bend from waist to the left and then to the right.	18	20 ea. side	25 ea. side
Warm-Up Waist Thighs Legs	7	**Running in Place:** Stand tall and run in place, lifting legs high. If you cannot jog or run, march in place. Easy does it.	34	40 sec.	45 sec.
Hips Thighs	8	**Half Squats:** Hold on to a chair; bend knees, pause, straighten to standing position.	28	15	20
Legs	9	**Toe Raises:** Raise up on toes, hold for one count, and lower to original position.	32	20	25
Shoulders Arms Waist	10	**The Swimmer:** Bend over at waist, bend knees, bring arm up to ear, and pretend you are swimming.	64	40 sec.	50 sec.
Waist Arms Back	11	**Cobra Stretch:** Lie on floor or bed, then lift upper body with your arms; arch back, head up.	98	8	10
Warm-Down	12	**Rag Doll Relaxer:** Bend at waist while keeping back flat; arms hang loosely toward floor.	62	15 sec.	20 sec.

Problem Zone Fitness Program—Level 1

Exercise	Problem Area(s)	Week 1 Goal	Week 1 Actual	Week 2 Goal	Week 2 Actual	Week 3 Goal	Week 3 Actual	Week 4 Goal	Week 4 Actual
	Warm-Up Exercises								
	Neck & Chin								
	Chest								
	Back								
	Arms (Back & Front)								
	Shoulders								
	Waist & Stomach								
	Hips								
	Thighs								
	Lower Legs								

Exercise Level 2

Congratulations! You have obviously become comfortable with Exercise Level 1, so it is time to change your program and try out Level 2.

Level 2 is similar to Level 1 in that it features the Daily Dozen exercises designed to build muscle strength and endurance, while also improving the most important single muscle in the body—the heart. The difference is that the exercises are slightly more strenuous and they generally feature more reps. I have made use of the same warm-up exercise, Dynamic Swings, for all three levels because it is a terrific overall muscle worker. When you create your own programs (either for problem zones or at a level beyond Level 3), you might want to use a warm-up that is even a bit more strenuous than the Dynamic Swings: perhaps Punching or Windmills.

Remember that as you get into your Level 2 program, you are not required to stay there. If you get into it and begin to feel that it is too difficult, either drop back to Level 1 or decrease the reps I have suggested. Check your heart rate. If you are unable to properly perform a specific exercise, but want to stay in Level 2, do only one rep or skip the exercise entirely until you feel you are physically ready for it. Always strive to do one more rep, but don't overdo it. I can recall the first time I did Leg Lunges. I said to Jack, "Oh, this is easy . . ." *Wow!* Did I learn fast! I did more than I should have and suffered the next few days with sore muscles in my thighs (both inner and outer). You see, my inner thigh muscles had not been worked for a long time. That's why it is always important to *make haste slowly*, making sure that your muscles are getting their share of work.

Now that you are farther along with your program of exercise, I'd like to share a few more hints with you:

1. **Wear something comfortable so as not to restrict your movements.**

2. **Keep a small rug or exercise mat handy for floor exercises.**

3. **Before starting your program, do a little stretching.** Try to touch the ceiling or try to climb a wall until you feel more limber.

4. **Be sure you are performing the exercises correctly.** Think into the area you are working. For example, if you are exercising the back of the arms, think into the tricep muscle. Movements must be full and complete. The more you concentrate, the better the results.

5. **Never hold your breath while exercising.**

6. **Exercise on a regular basis.** By that I mean every day or at least six days a week.

7. **Don't make excuses.** One excuse leads to another and pretty soon you've dropped your exercise program. Remember, you are never too busy to do the things you really want to do.

8. **Many people ask the question: "When is the best time to exercise?"** There is really no set time; some people prefer to exercise upon rising, others before they go to bed. But do not exercise within an hour after a meal. Do make your exercising a regular part of your day.

9. **If you have access to a mirror while exercising, it helps to see if you are doing the exercise correctly.**

10. **Use resistance as much as possible.** For example, the books and canned goods I've suggested can provide the necessary added resistance. The more resistance, the quicker the results. If you are unable to attend an exercise facility with special exercise equipment, this is the next best alternative.

11. **Constantly check your posture.** As we get older, we all have a tendency to slump. It's simply gravity catching up with us. Stand tall, shoulders back, head erect. Feel like a string is attached to your ears and is pulling you up straight. As it turns out, the old idea of walking with a book on your head is an excellent way to practice good posture.

12. **Breathe deeply, inhale through your nose, exhale through your mouth.**

Keep with Level 2, but remember that you should not rush through it in an attempt to reach Level 3 before you're ready for it. It will always be waiting there for you, always ready to work for you to further your fitness.

Week 1 and 2

Area Affected	Daily Dozen	Exercise and Description	Page Ref.	Week 1 Repetitions	Week 2 Repetitions
Overall Warm-Up	1	**Dynamic Swings:** Swing down through legs and up again. Depending on strength condition, use light book or 3-lb. dumbell between hands.	2	15	18
Neck Shoulders	2	**Neck Rotator:** Stand in a wide stance and bend forward at the waist with hands on knees. Try to look at ceiling; turn head slowly from side to side.	68	6 ea. side	8 ea. side
Waist Arms	3	**Windmills:** Bend at waist, right arm stretched out. Simultaneously swing right arm across body and try to touch left hand to ceiling. Swing back, alternating with opposite hands.	106	5 sec.	10 sec.
Shoulders Waist	4	**Knees into Chest** (Sitting): Sit on edge of chair and bring one or both knees into chest. Keep knees together when lifting both legs. **Bicycle:** Pump your legs as you would riding a bicycle.	76 78 82	5 10 sec.	10 15 sec.
Hips Thighs	5	**Leg Lunges to the Side:** Hold on to chair for balance. Lunge to the right with right leg, step back and lunge to the left on left leg.	26	3 ea. side	6 ea. side
Shoulders	6	**Posture Stretch:** Arms open, feet wide apart, head up and to the back slightly. Try to crush imaginary walnut between shoulder blades.	118	5	10
Arms	7	**Back Arm Extension:** Bend at waist holding weights, elbows high. Extend arms back toward ceiling. **Front Arm Curl:** Hold weight in both hands. Curl lower arms from elbow toward face.	88 92	3 5	5 10
Hips Thighs	8	**Leg Extensions** (3-way variation): Stand erect, point toe, extend right leg to back as far as possible, then out to side as far as possible. Now flex foot and cross same leg over in front of opposite leg.	24	10 ea. leg	15 ea. leg
Chest	9	**Supine Press:** Lie on back, knees up. Use a book in each hand (or 3-lb. weights). Lift books to ceiling, then bring down smoothly to shoulders.	94	10	15
Chest Arms	10	**Push-Ups:** Push upper body off floor until arms are fully extended. Lower and repeat.	36	As many as possible	As many as possible
Waist	11	**Sit-Ups to Feet:** On back, hands above head, legs in air, two feet apart; try to sit up, bringing hands between legs. Variation: Lie on floor, put feet in chair and try to sit up.	42	As many as possible	As many as possible
Legs Thighs	12	**Leg Curls:** Lie on floor, face down; reach out with hands in front of you as far as possible. Bring lower legs up from knees; hold for count of one; return.	96	5	8

Week 3 and 4

Area Affected	Daily Dozen	Exercise and Description	Page Ref.	Week 3 Repetitions	Week 4 Repetitions
Overall Warm-Up	1	**Dynamic Swings:** Swing down through legs and up again. Depending on strength condition, use light book or 3-lb. dumbell between hands.	2	20	25
Neck Shoulders	2	**Neck Rotator:** Stand in a wide stance and bend forward at the waist with hands on knees. Try to look at ceiling; turn head slowly from side to side.	68	10 ea. side	12 ea. side
Waist Arms	3	**Windmills:** Bend at waist, right arm stretched out. Simultaneously swing right arm across body and try to touch left hand to ceiling. Swing back, alternating with opposite hands.	106	15 sec.	20 sec.
Shoulders Waist	4	**Knees into Chest** (Sitting): Sit on edge of chair and bring one or both knees into chest. Keep knees together when lifting both legs. **Bicycle:** Pump your legs as you would riding a bicycle.	76 78 82	12 20 sec.	15 30 sec.
Hips Thighs	5	**Leg Lunges to the Side:** Hold on to chair for balance. Lunge to the right with right leg, step back and lunge to the left on left leg.	26	12 ea. side	15 ea. side
Shoulders	6	**Posture Stretch:** Arms open, feet wide apart, head up and to the back slightly. Try to crush imaginary walnut between shoulder blades.	118	15	20
Arms	7	**Back Arm Extension:** Bend at waist holding weights, elbows high. Extend arms back toward ceiling. **Front Arm Curl:** Hold weight in both hands. Curl lower arms from elbow toward face.	88 92	8 15	10 20
Hips Thighs	8	**Leg Extensions** (3-way variation): Stand erect, point toe, extend right leg to back as far as possible, then out to side as far as possible. Now flex foot and cross same leg over in front of opposite leg.	24	20 ea. leg	25 ea. leg
Chest	9	**Supine Press:** Lie on back, knees up. Use a book in each hand (or 3-lb. weights). Lift books to ceiling, then bring down smoothly to shoulders.	94	20	25
Chest Arms	10	**Push-Ups:** Push upper body off floor until arms are fully extended. Lower and repeat.	36	As many as possible	As many as possible
Waist	11	**Sit-Ups to Feet:** On back, hands above head, legs in air, two feet apart; try to sit up, bringing hands between legs. Variation: Lie on floor, put feet in chair and try to sit up.	42	As many as possible	As many as possible
Legs Thighs	12	**Leg Curls:** Lie on floor, face down; reach out with hands in front of you as far as possible. Bring lower legs up from knees; hold for count of one; return.	96	10	12

Problem Zone Fitness Program—Level 2

Exercise	Problem Area(s)	Week 1 Goal	Week 1 Actual	Week 2 Goal	Week 2 Actual	Week 3 Goal	Week 3 Actual	Week 4 Goal	Week 4 Actual
	Warm-Up Exercises								
	Neck & Chin								
	Chest								
	Back								
	Arms (Back & Front)								
	Shoulders								
	Waist & Stomach								
	Hips								
	Thighs								
	Lower Legs								

Exercise Level 3

Congratulations are once again in order. You have worked steadily on making regular exercise a part of your life, and have reached Level 3. Certainly, doing *no* exercise can be a part of a person's life, and for too many people it is, but you have overcome that barrier and you are well on your way...

Level 3 is in all ways a more advanced level. Yet it maintains the same format as Levels 1 and 2. The Daily Dozen exercises are there, and there is a page of fill-ins for problem zones. You'll find that the exercises at this level are somewhat more ambitious, strenuous, or have more reps. Level 3 should be done only afer successfully negotiating the other two levels. Again, don't be concerned if you need to drop back to a previous level if you feel overly tired or strained. It is also not necessary for you to remain at Level 3 continuously. Try going back to Level 1 or 2 and increasing the reps or weight. Another way to change is to create another level: Level 4, Level 5, etc.— designed by you, designed for you. If you do this each month, you could end up with a dozen levels covering the entire year—and forming a chronicle of your progress. The secret is to continue to change your program for best results. I have not listed every exercise that I know, but these are some of the best basic exercises I've encountered. Feel free to add others, but be certain that you know just what area the exercise is working.

Remember that it is a myth that older means weaker. It was reported in the very first issue of the University of California, Berkeley, *Wellness Letter*, that some types of strength remain nearly constant throughout life. Authorities on the subject of fitness support the fact that regular exercise can help prevent degenerative disease and slow down deterioration due to aging. In other words, you can help slow or stop the aging process through exercise. So don't be surprised if by the time you reach Level 3 you have noticed more energy and strength. You'll probably find, also, that you are sleeping better and waking up more refreshed, with more energy for work and play.

There is often more truth than fiction when it comes to cliches. I have listed some of those to which I adhere:

1. **Use it or lose it.** If you don't use your muscles, you will lose them. The more you use your body, the more it improves.

2. **People don't wear out, they rust out.** Slow deterioration and not being able to do what we want to do are our fears as we age. Like a rusty door hinge, we slow down and creak—but exercise is like oil to our rusty bodies.

3. **Treat your body as your closest friend.** I certainly wouldn't want to abuse my closest friend.

4. **The more you do, the more you can do.** This is called the Training Effect and is just as true for an Olympic athlete as it is for the least active among us.

5. **Practice makes perfect.** We all know this one. All we have to do is to look at someone who can play the piano. Without practice, there is no music.

If you follow the hints and suggestions in all three levels, you'll have earned the right to enjoy the fit lifestyle...a lifestyle that has no age barriers.

Week 1 and 2

Area Affected	Daily Dozen	Exercise and Description	Page Ref.	Week 1 Repetitions	Week 2 Repetitions
Overall Warm-Up	1	**Dynamic Swings:** Swing down through legs and up again. Depending on strength condition, use heavy book or 5–10-lb. dumbell between hands.	2	15	18
Waist	2	**Sit-Ups to Feet:** See Level 2, Exercise 11, or: **Jack Knife:** Extend hands behind head; lift legs and body simultaneously. Try to touch toes with hands.	42 102	As many as possible	As many as possible
Back Thighs Hips	3	**Arch Ups:** Lie flat on back, arms by sides for support. Bend knees while feet are flat; raise up hips as high as possible.	72	5	8
Chest	4	**Push-Ups:** See Level 2, Exercise 10, or: **Standard Push-Ups:** Lie flat, legs together. Rise up on your toes; push body off floor so weight rests on hands and toes.	36 74	As many as possible	As many as possible
Waist	5	**Knee into Chest** (called Donkey Kicks): On hands and knees, head down, try to touch your right knee to your nose. Extend leg to back, arching back while looking toward ceiling. Repeat with other leg.	38	6	12
Chest	6	**Pullovers:** Lie on bench or over armless chair. Place book between hands, keeping arms straight. Let book pull arms over as far as possible; then pull book over chest.	84	6	12
Shoulders Arms	7	**Lateral Raises:** Hold weights (canned goods) out to sides of body. Keeping arms straight, raise arms over head.	86	5	8
Hips Thighs	8	**Hip, Thigh Lift:** On floor, lie on side; use lower arm to support head. Raise upper leg, keeping it straight. Bring lower leg up to meet upper leg; hold two seconds. Alternate legs.	104	3	6
Overall Exercise	9	**Punching:** Bend slightly at the knees. Pretend you are hitting a punching bag. Try to hit the wall behind you with your elbow, then punch out at the wall in front of you trying to hit it.	112	5 sec.	8 sec.
Hips Thighs	10	**Forward Leg Lunges:** Put hands on hips or hold on to chair for balance. Lunge forward similar to a fencing pose; step back and lunge on opposite leg.	58	5 each side	8 each side
Waist Legs Thighs Warm-down	11	**Running in Place:** Do not run with your legs behind you—keep them under you. For best results, run by lifting your knees high. Great cardiovascular workout.	34	Knees high 10 sec.	Knees high 20 sec.
Hips Thighs	12	**Duck Walk:** Bend knees into a half squat; lean body slightly to the back (like a lean-to). Walk forward and backward like a duck.	28	10 sec.	20 sec.

Week 3 and 4

Area Affected	Daily Dozen	Exercise and Description	Page Ref.	Week 3 Repetitions	Week 4 Repetitions
Overall Warm-Up	1	**Dynamic Swings:** Swing down through legs and up again. Depending on strength condition, use heavy book or 5–10-lb. dumbell between hands.	2	20	25
Waist	2	**Sit-Ups to Feet:** See Level 2, Exercise 11, or: **Jack Knife:** Extend hands behind head; lift legs and body simultaneously. Try to touch toes with hands.	42 102	As many as possible	As many as possible
Back Thighs Hips	3	**Arch Ups:** Lie flat on back, arms by sides for support. Bend knees while feet are flat; raise up hips as high as possible.	72	10	12
Chest	4	**Push-Ups:** See Level 2, Exercise 10, or: **Standard Push-Ups:** Lie flat, legs together. Rise up on your toes; push body off floor so weight rests on hands and toes.	36 74	As many as possible	As many as possible
Waist	5	**Knee into Chest** (called Donkey Kicks): On hands and knees, head down, try to touch your right knee to your nose. Extend leg to back, arching back while looking toward ceiling. Repeat with other leg.	38	15	20
Chest	6	**Pullovers:** Lie on bench or over armless chair. Place book between hands, keeping arms straight. Let book pull arms over as far as possible; then pull book over chest.	84	15	20
Shoulders Arms	7	**Lateral Raises:** Hold weights (canned goods) out to sides of body. Keeping arms straight, raise arms over head.	86	10	15
Hips Thighs	8	**Hip, Thigh Lift:** On floor, lie on side; use lower arm to support head. Raise upper leg, keeping it straight. Bring lower leg up to meet upper leg; hold two seconds. Alternate legs.	104	9	12
Overall Exercise	9	**Punching:** Bend slightly at the knees. Pretend you are hitting a punching bag. Try to hit the wall behind you with your elbow, then punch out at the wall in front of you trying to hit it.	112	10 sec.	12 sec.
Hips Thighs	10	**Forward Leg Lunges:** Put hands on hips or hold on to chair for balance. Lunge forward similar to a fencing pose; step back and lunge on opposite leg.	58	12 each side	15 each side
Waist Legs Thighs Warm-down	11	**Running in Place:** Do not run with your legs behind you—keep them under you. For best results, run by lifting your knees high. Great cardiovascular workout.	34	Knees high 30 sec.	Knees high 35 sec.
Hips Thighs	12	**Duck Walk:** Bend knees into a half squat; lean body slightly to the back (like a lean-to). Walk forward and backward like a duck.	28	30 sec.	35 sec.

Problem Zone Fitness Program—Level 3

Exercise	Problem Area(s)	Week 1 Goal	Week 1 Actual	Week 2 Goal	Week 2 Actual	Week 3 Goal	Week 3 Actual	Week 4 Goal	Week 4 Actual
	Warm-Up Exercises								
	Neck & Chin								
	Chest								
	Back								
	Arms (Back & Front)								
	Shoulders								
	Waist & Stomach								
	Hips								
	Thighs								
	Lower Legs								

"Before" and "After" photos

"One picture is worth a thousand words" is a statement that holds a lot of truth. I know a woman who committed herself to losing 100 pounds. To help her reach her goal, she had a picture of herself taken and then she pasted it on the door of the refrigerator. Every time she went to the refrigerator (through force of habit), she saw the picture, looked at it, and said to herself, "I don't want to look like that anymore." She immediately closed the door and let the snack go uneaten.

Within a year, she lost 100 pounds.

Now maybe you don't need to lose 100 pounds, but you do want to reshape your body into something resembling what you looked like when you were at your best. It's a well-known fact that through proper nutrition and exercise you can help retard the aging process. Remember, practically every cell in your body changes every 90 days, so it stands to reason if you start today on a regular exercise routine and proper nutrition, in 90 days you are well on your way to a new you.

I can understand how many people would be motivated to get into fitness for the sole purpose of restructuring themselves. But I find that the shape and contours your body enjoys as a gift from being fit are very much secondary to the joys of fitness itself. Certainly, it's nice to have people look surprised when I tell them how old I am. But that's not my main reason for maintaining a fitness lifestyle.

I'm not saying that wanting to reshape your body into something resembling what it looked like when you were at your best isn't a workable motivating factor. It most certainly is. I've repeatedly found, however, that people who take up fitness to attempt to move the clock back to find that younger body they feel lurks within them usually end up admitting that the reason they keep at fitness is that they've really become hooked on it, that it makes them feel better, and that it enhances their lives.

My feeling is that *anything* that gets you involved in fitness is a good thing.

I predict, however, that if you initially get interested in fitness to trim down or in some way redesign your figure, you'll eventually change your priorities—and your initial concern for your "new" figure will take care of itself as you further pursue your future in fitness.

I do feel that what you physically look like is the outward glow of fitness. And I feel that being able to see some progress in reshaping your body can be a very real barometer of your progress.

Toward this end, I've created a space in the Appendix of this book where you can place a photograph of yourself as you embark on this year's worth of fitness and a place for a photo of what you physically look like 52 weeks later.

What you should do for these two photos is take a photograph of yourself (if your camera has a timing device) at the start of your fitness year, and another one year later. If you cannot take the photo yourself, have a good friend push the button for you. Shoot both photographs at the same location, with the same camera, and use the same pose. I suggest that if you are serious about this, you take the photo in a swimsuit. For females, it should be in a two-piece, so that you'll be able to see the development in your stomach muscles after a year's worth of workouts; for males, use swimming trunks or briefs.

Don't flex. Merely stand facing the camera, spread your feet about 18 inches, and place your fists on your hips. You want to see progress in a relaxed pose, not in one that's bulging with pumped-up muscles.

Your goals in fitness (which you're writing down in each week's appropriate block) may be to firm up that stomach area. Believe me, after a year's work, you will see very apparent differences. The same goes for your thighs and your upper arms. Make an extra print of your "before" and "after" photos and send me a set and tell me about your progress.

About the remainder of the Appendix

We've already discussed, briefly, the inclusion of the four season meals which are contained in the Appendix of this book. Besides providing good, simple, nourishing meals, they provide a centerpiece for your evaluation of goals, while giving you a perfect time to review your accomplishments to that point. Think of it as a celebration feast. Enjoy it and use it every three months as the pivotal point of your fitness program as it takes one giant step after the other.

We've also discussed the ''before'' and ''after'' photograph of yourself as a great way of keeping track of your progress. Once you have three or four years of diaries filled in, your going back through the ''before'' and ''after'' pages should be a real treat.

So what else is lurking back there in the Appendix?

Aerobic Sports Guide. My feeling about exercising and fitness is that it's more fun if it's being done as play. And fitness can certainly be made closer to play if you are securing your fitness through doing some sport. The only sports that offer true fitness are those that promote cardiovascular fitness. These are called aerobic sports. You'll see the most common ones listed on pages 144 and 145. I can't stress enough how important those sports are as roadways to complete fitness. They are excellent, also, because you can do every one of them by yourself, with friends, or you can compete in most of them if you are so inclined.

I should stress, of course, that an overall fitness program extends beyond these sports. It includes good nutrition and adequate sleep; it avoids bad habits such as smoking; and it involves additional exercise to develop parts of your body that some of the aerobic sports do not develop. Running, for instance, is excellent for building cardiovascular fitness and for building strong legs; but it doesn't do much to build the upper body. For instance, if you take up running to stay fit, supplement it with a regular program of building your upper body strength.

Calories Burned Chart. Everyone seems to be obsessed with calories. This chart is fun. It gives the number of calories burned while engaging in various activities, both of an everyday nature and activities that are fitness-related. It is so much better to help rid yourself of unwanted calories by exercising them away than it is by strictly dieting. Dieting does nothing to tone your body as you lose weight. If you merely diet, and are successful, you can potentially look worse after you've lost the weight than you did when you were heavy, simply because your skin seems to hang loose.

So get rid of your weight by exercising and watching those calories. You'll more easily reach the goals you have for yourself that way, and that ''after'' picture will more accurately reflect the person you would like to be. Keep in mind, too, that exercising can be worked into things you might have to do around the house. You can work so many little exercising things into your daily life. Going shopping? Is the store within a mile of home? Then leave the car keys where they are and walk to the store and back. If it's a mile out and a mile back, that's 200 calories burned just like that.

The Questionnaire. I've included a questionnaire about your fitness. If you'd like to fill it out and send it in to me, I'd certainly appreciate it. I'd like to know a little bit more about you and your fitness goals. By knowing you better, I can customize my fitness crusade toward your needs. If you want to tell me more about your fitness than is reflected in the questionnaire, please feel free to enclose a letter. I'd love to hear from you.

How to properly take measurements

Everything to do with losing or gaining weight is predicated on the scale.

I feel the scale is important, but I feel the tape measure is even more important because it tells you what your physical condition is. The scale can't tell you what kind of improvement you have made to your body. Proportion is of utmost importance. A lot of people talk about losing or gaining weight as their ultimate goal, but what they really want is good proportions: the ratio of chest to waist to hips, etc.

Everyone can be well proportioned if they work at it. Think of yourself as a piece of sculpture. My husband has a pinch test he uses. Pinch the side of your waist and if you find an inch of fat there, you're liable to be 10 pounds overweight.

When I met Jack LaLanne, I was underweight but fat. My measurements were 33-27-33, and I weighed 107 pounds. Through exercise and proper nutrition I reproportioned my body to what I am today: 36-25-36, at 117 pounds. Exercise reproportioned my body and proper nutrition helped me assimilate my food properly.

I have maintained those proportions and that weight for the last 30 years after changing a few bad habits for good. Remember that exercise is a body normalizer. What this means is that if you are underweight, it will help build you up, and if you're overweight, it will help trim you down. I was an under-exerciser and an assimilator of junk food—a junk food junkie. But regular exercise and good food turned me around.

So what happens when you embark on an exercise program? The fat begins to melt off, to be replaced by...muscle. And what do we know about muscle? Right. It weighs more than fat. So you may look at yourself after 10 weeks of exercise and careful attention to good food, and say, ''Gee, I look better, but every time I step onto the scale, my heart stops when I see how much weight I've *gained*.''

What's happened is that you've gained weight because you've replaced fat with muscle. And there's nothing wrong with that, although your bathroom scale may try to tell you that there is.

So don't become obsessed with your (height relative to your) weight. Some of those tables that dictate weight ranges for various heights are obsolete. What you should weigh is what is right for you, what allows you to be healthy and happy.

So where does that leave us, and what's my point, right?

Scales lie. Remember that first and foremost. So it leaves us taking *measurements* of ourselves, and ignoring the scales.

On the next pages you'll see some blown up photographs of taking measurements of your body parts. Important places like the waist and stomach and calves and ankles and chest. Measure yourself very carefully, and follow the instructions for each measurement exactly. Then jot the measurements (to the quarter-of-an-inch) in the appropriate places on page xliii.

This is your starting point for this year of fitness. At the end of every four-week period, there'll be a two-page section where you'll be asked to take your measurements again. There is a page on the left that reviews the places to measure in somewhat smaller pictures than on the next two pages, and on the right page there are empty blocks just like there are on page xliii. Take your measurements faithfully and keep track of them. Always take the measurements at the same time of day. I suggest when you get up in the morning.

These numbers are so much more important than the numbers you see on your bathroom scale that it's difficult for me to make the point strongly enough.

And don't get discouraged because you don't see radical changes in your measurements within the first measuring period. Keep in mind that it is unhealthy to have your body go through extremely rapid changes.

Your basic statistics at the end of the year will indicate you're a new person.

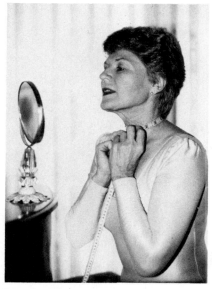

Neck. Using a tape measure and a mirror so that you can accurately see the readings, wrap the measure snugly around your neck, at the point where the male Adam's apple is located.

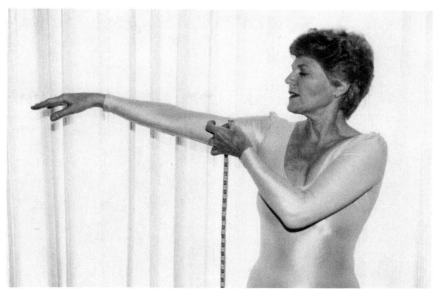

Upper Arm. This is a real problem area for some women, because when they hold their arm out parallel to the ground, the underside of the arm sags. This condition can be minimized by exercising. Make your measurement around the muscle that pops up on bodybuilders when you say, "Make a muscle."

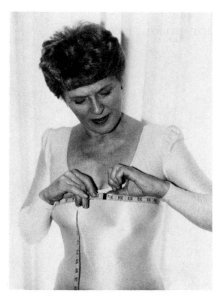

Bust. Run the tape around your back and bring it around and across your bust, measuring it on the most ample portion. Make sure that the tape around your back is cinched up properly.

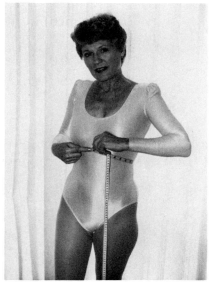

Midriff. Slide the tape down from your bust to your midriff, which is directly under your breasts, along the side of your rib cage. Make sure the tape is taut and take a reading to the nearest quarter inch.

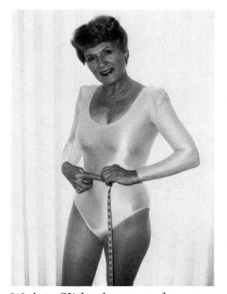

Waist. Slide the tape down even farther, until it is around your waist, which should be the narrowest portion of your trunk. This is a critical measurement for many women. Make it accurate.

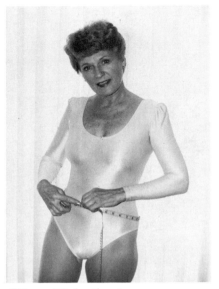

Hips. Slide the tape measure down even farther. The hips are the widest portion of your trunk below your waist. A measurement of the hips will also include measuring the stomach, so this one's important.

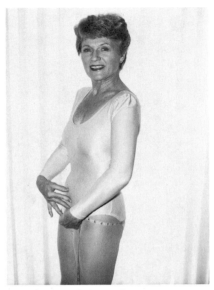

Buttocks. Bring the tape down even farther, sliding it around your buttocks at the widest section you can locate. Make sure that the entire tape is even and totally parallel to the ground or you'll get inaccuracies.

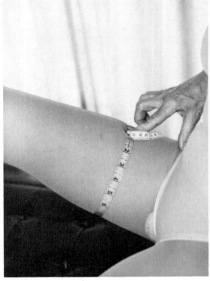

Upper thigh. Take these next four measurements while sitting down. Wrap the tape around your upper thigh at a point three or four inches down from the juncture of leg to trunk.

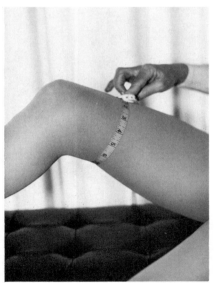

Lower thigh. Wrap the tape around your lower thigh at a point about three or four inches up from your knee. Don't flex your leg muscles when doing this. Allow them to be relaxed.

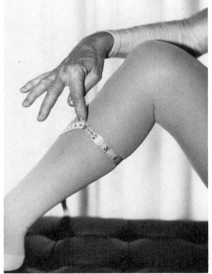

Calf. Measure at the widest point around your calf muscle, but don't flex the muscle while you're doing so. This is the most closely-packed muscle mass in the entire body.

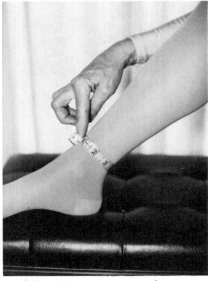

Ankle. Measure just above your ankle bones. This measurement may seem trivial, but it can be a real indicator of whether or not you are retaining water. Proper exercise and diet can slim down and tone up the ankle.

Your monthly body measurements

Record your measurements from the first check of your body parts in the boxes below of that part from pages xli and xlii. This is your starting point for this year's fitness. Each month you'll have a review of these measurements and a place in which to record your progress.

Neck

Upper Arm

Bust

Midriff

Waist

Hips

Buttocks

Upper thigh

Lower thigh

Calf

Ankle

A Year's Worth
of Fitness

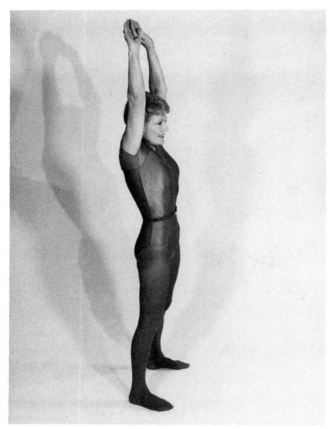

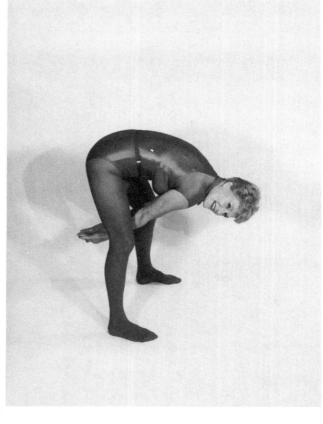

Dynamic Swings
Exercising on a regular basis is essential to the success of any fitness program. It is also essential that you think into the particular muscle you are exercising. The Dynamic Swing is a wonderful all-over warm-up exercise. Stand with feet shoulder-width apart; reach as high as possible overhead, stretching slightly to the back—swing smoothly down through your legs and back up again. Bend your knees slightly.

Goals for this week:

1. _____

2. _____

Goals for this month:

1. _____

2. _____

Take your life into your own hands and wring the most from it. By doing that, you'll strengthen your life— and your hands.

Avocado and Tuna Sandwich
3 oz. of water pack tuna
¼ of large avocado (or ½ of small or medium avocado)

Mash tuna and avocado, and spread on sandwich with lettuce.

This week covers _____ , _____ , _____ , **to** _____ , _____ , _____ .
          month   day   year   month   day   year

| **Monday** | E X E R C I S E | Activity _____
 _____
 Time _____
 Distance _____
 Pace _____
 Effort: ☐ Easy   ☐ Moderate
         ☐ Hard   ☐ Extreme | Remarks (fitness): _____
 _____

 Remarks (personal): _____
 _____
 _____ |
| **Resting Pulse Rate** / **Weight At Rising** | | | |

| **Tuesday** | E X E R C I S E | Activity _____
 _____
 Time _____
 Distance _____
 Pace _____
 Effort: ☐ Easy   ☐ Moderate
         ☐ Hard   ☐ Extreme | Remarks (fitness): _____
 _____

 Remarks (personal): _____
 _____
 _____ |
| **Resting Pulse Rate** / **Weight At Rising** | | | |

| **Wednesday** | E X E R C I S E | Activity _____
 _____
 Time _____
 Distance _____
 Pace _____
 Effort: ☐ Easy   ☐ Moderate
         ☐ Hard   ☐ Extreme | Remarks (fitness): _____
 _____

 Remarks (personal): _____
 _____
 _____ |
| **Resting Pulse Rate** / **Weight At Rising** | | | |

| **Thursday** | E X E R C I S E | Activity _____
 _____
 Time _____
 Distance _____
 Pace _____
 Effort: ☐ Easy   ☐ Moderate
         ☐ Hard   ☐ Extreme | Remarks (fitness): _____
 _____

 Remarks (personal): _____
 _____
 _____ |
| **Resting Pulse Rate** / **Weight At Rising** | | | |

| **Friday** | E X E R C I S E | Activity _____
 _____
 Time _____
 Distance _____
 Pace _____
 Effort: ☐ Easy   ☐ Moderate
         ☐ Hard   ☐ Extreme | Remarks (fitness): _____
 _____

 Remarks (personal): _____
 _____
 _____ |
| **Resting Pulse Rate** / **Weight At Rising** | | | |

| **Saturday** | E X E R C I S E | Activity _____
 _____
 Time _____
 Distance _____
 Pace _____
 Effort: ☐ Easy   ☐ Moderate
         ☐ Hard   ☐ Extreme | Remarks (fitness): _____
 _____

 Remarks (personal): _____
 _____
 _____ |
| **Resting Pulse Rate** / **Weight At Rising** | | | |

| **Sunday** | E X E R C I S E | Activity _____
 _____
 Time _____
 Distance _____
 Pace _____
 Effort: ☐ Easy   ☐ Moderate
         ☐ Hard   ☐ Extreme | Remarks (fitness): _____
 _____

 Remarks (personal): _____
 _____
 _____ |
| **Resting Pulse Rate** / **Weight At Rising** | | | |

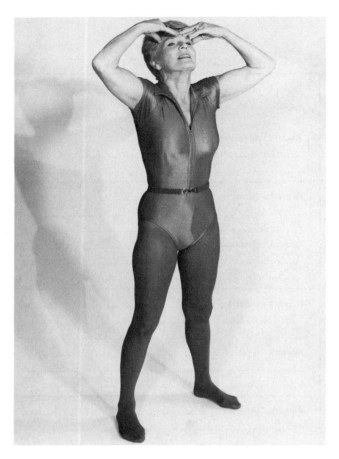

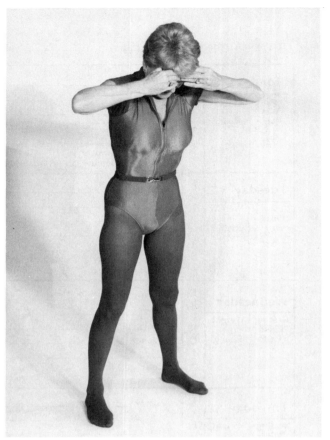

Neck and Chin Firmer
This exercise is terrific for the chin and neck-line. Stand or sit erect. Place your fingers on your forehead. Now try to put your chin on your chest resisting with your fingers. Then bring your head back up as far as possible, resisting with your neck.

Goals for this week:
1. _____
2. _____
Goals for this month:
1. _____
2. _____

Bean Sprout Salad
2 cups fresh bean sprouts
1 cup celery, sliced thin
1 cup radishes, sliced thin
4 scallions, sliced
Dressing:
¾ cup oil
⅛ cup vinegar
¼ cup soy sauce

Mix together oil, vinegar and soy sauce. Pour over vegetables. However, do not use entire amount, as it may be too much for this amount of vegetables; this depends on your taste.

The first two months of a fitness program are an uphill battle; after that, it's all gentle coasting.

This week covers _____ , _____ , _____ , to _____ , _____ , _____ .
month   day   year   month   day   year

Monday

Resting Pulse Rate	Weight At Rising

E X E R C I S E

Activity _____
_____
Time _____
Distance _____
Pace _____
Effort: ☐ Easy ☐ Moderate ☐ Hard ☐ Extreme

Remarks (fitness): _____
_____
Remarks (personal): _____
_____
_____

Tuesday

Resting Pulse Rate	Weight At Rising

E X E R C I S E

Activity _____
_____
Time _____
Distance _____
Pace _____
Effort: ☐ Easy ☐ Moderate ☐ Hard ☐ Extreme

Remarks (fitness): _____
_____
Remarks (personal): _____
_____

Wednesday

Resting Pulse Rate	Weight At Rising

E X E R C I S E

Activity _____
_____
Time _____
Distance _____
Pace _____
Effort: ☐ Easy ☐ Moderate ☐ Hard ☐ Extreme

Remarks (fitness): _____
_____
Remarks (personal): _____
_____

Thursday

Resting Pulse Rate	Weight At Rising

E X E R C I S E

Activity _____
_____
Time _____
Distance _____
Pace _____
Effort: ☐ Easy ☐ Moderate ☐ Hard ☐ Extreme

Remarks (fitness): _____
_____
Remarks (personal): _____
_____

Friday

Resting Pulse Rate	Weight At Rising

E X E R C I S E

Activity _____
_____
Time _____
Distance _____
Pace _____
Effort: ☐ Easy ☐ Moderate ☐ Hard ☐ Extreme

Remarks (fitness): _____
_____
Remarks (personal): _____
_____

Saturday

Resting Pulse Rate	Weight At Rising

E X E R C I S E

Activity _____
_____
Time _____
Distance _____
Pace _____
Effort: ☐ Easy ☐ Moderate ☐ Hard ☐ Extreme

Remarks (fitness): _____
_____
Remarks (personal): _____
_____

Sunday

Resting Pulse Rate	Weight At Rising

E X E R C I S E

Activity _____
_____
Time _____
Distance _____
Pace _____
Effort: ☐ Easy ☐ Moderate ☐ Hard ☐ Extreme

Remarks (fitness): _____
_____
Remarks (personal): _____
_____

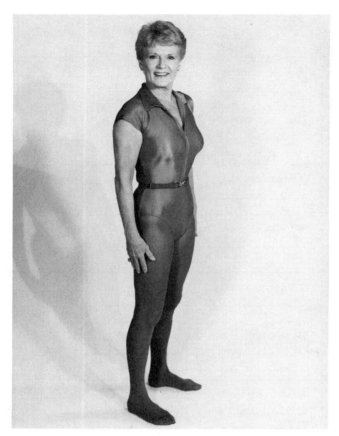

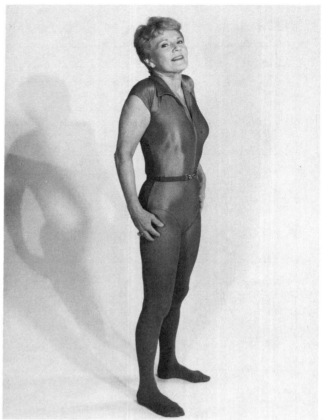

Shoulder Shrugs
The Shoulder Shrug is terrific if you suffer from stiffness in the neck and shoulders, especially if it is due to tension. Stand straight, feet shoulder-width apart; allow your shoulders to shrug. Now, bring your shoulders up toward your ears, hold for a count of three, and relax them again.

If you're worried about stress in your life, it probably means that there's something to worry about. So do something physical about it today.

Goals for this week:
1. _____
2. _____

Goals for this month:
1. _____
2. _____

Lemon-Orange Spicy Drink

3 oranges	1 tsp. whole cloves
2 lemons	1 cup honey
6 cups water	
stick of cinnamon	

Squeeze the juice and set it aside. Coarsely chop the rinds and combine with water, spices and honey in a 2- or 3-quart saucepan. Boil for 5 minutes and strain into pitcher. Discard rinds and spices. Let cool and add the juices. Chill. May also be served hot.

This week covers _____ , _____ , _____ , to _____ , _____ , _____ .
          month   day   year   month   day   year

Monday

Resting Pulse Rate	Weight At Rising

EXERCISE

Activity _____
_____
Time _____
Distance _____
Pace _____
Effort: ☐ Easy ☐ Moderate ☐ Hard ☐ Extreme

Remarks (fitness): _____
_____
_____
Remarks (personal): _____
_____
_____

Tuesday

Resting Pulse Rate	Weight At Rising

EXERCISE

Activity _____
_____
Time _____
Distance _____
Pace _____
Effort: ☐ Easy ☐ Moderate ☐ Hard ☐ Extreme

Remarks (fitness): _____
_____
_____
Remarks (personal): _____
_____
_____

Wednesday

Resting Pulse Rate	Weight At Rising

EXERCISE

Activity _____
_____
Time _____
Distance _____
Pace _____
Effort: ☐ Easy ☐ Moderate ☐ Hard ☐ Extreme

Remarks (fitness): _____
_____
_____
Remarks (personal): _____
_____
_____

Thursday

Resting Pulse Rate	Weight At Rising

EXERCISE

Activity _____
_____
Time _____
Distance _____
Pace _____
Effort: ☐ Easy ☐ Moderate ☐ Hard ☐ Extreme

Remarks (fitness): _____
_____
_____
Remarks (personal): _____
_____
_____

Friday

Resting Pulse Rate	Weight At Rising

EXERCISE

Activity _____
_____
Time _____
Distance _____
Pace _____
Effort: ☐ Easy ☐ Moderate ☐ Hard ☐ Extreme

Remarks (fitness): _____
_____
_____
Remarks (personal): _____
_____
_____

Saturday

Resting Pulse Rate	Weight At Rising

EXERCISE

Activity _____
_____
Time _____
Distance _____
Pace _____
Effort: ☐ Easy ☐ Moderate ☐ Hard ☐ Extreme

Remarks (fitness): _____
_____
_____
Remarks (personal): _____
_____
_____

Sunday

Resting Pulse Rate	Weight At Rising

EXERCISE

Activity _____
_____
Time _____
Distance _____
Pace _____
Effort: ☐ Easy ☐ Moderate ☐ Hard ☐ Extreme

Remarks (fitness): _____
_____
_____
Remarks (personal): _____
_____
_____

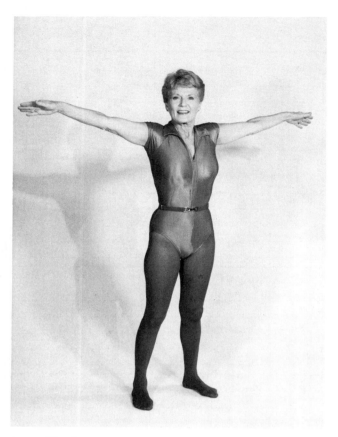

Fitness is the only valuable item you'll ever own that puts more back the more you take out of it.

Goals for this week:

1. _____

2. _____

Goals for this month:

1. _____

2. _____

Arm Circles

Arm circles help relieve nervous tension in the back of the neck and shoulder blades. They also help improve posture. Stand with your legs together or shoulder-width apart. Bring your arms out perpendicular to your sides and make circles with your hands, palms down.

Cheese and Spinach Squares

2 or 3 eggs
6 tbsp. whole wheat flour
1 lb. (2 cups) cottage cheese
½ lb. (2 cups) grated cheddar cheese
1 lb. fresh spinach
3 tbsp. wheat germ

Beat eggs, add flour, cottage cheese, and cheddar cheese in large bowl. Beat until smooth. Tear or chop spinach in bite-size pieces and add to mixture. Pour into well greased baking dish, approximately 8x12, and sprinkle with wheat germ. Bake uncovered at 350 degrees for approximately 45 minutes. Cut into squares for servings. *Variation:* Pour in pie plate; bake and serve as crustless quiche.

This week covers _____ , _____ , _____ , to _____ , _____ , _____ .
                       month   day   year   month   day   year

Monday

Resting Pulse Rate	Weight At Rising

EXERCISE

Activity _____
_____
Time _____
Distance _____
Pace _____
Effort: ☐ Easy ☐ Moderate
         ☐ Hard ☐ Extreme

Remarks (fitness): _____
_____
Remarks (personal): _____
_____

Tuesday

Resting Pulse Rate	Weight At Rising

EXERCISE

Activity _____
_____
Time _____
Distance _____
Pace _____
Effort: ☐ Easy ☐ Moderate
         ☐ Hard ☐ Extreme

Remarks (fitness): _____
_____
Remarks (personal): _____
_____

Wednesday

Resting Pulse Rate	Weight At Rising

EXERCISE

Activity _____
_____
Time _____
Distance _____
Pace _____
Effort: ☐ Easy ☐ Moderate
         ☐ Hard ☐ Extreme

Remarks (fitness): _____
_____
Remarks (personal): _____
_____

Thursday

Resting Pulse Rate	Weight At Rising

EXERCISE

Activity _____
_____
Time _____
Distance _____
Pace _____
Effort: ☐ Easy ☐ Moderate
         ☐ Hard ☐ Extreme

Remarks (fitness): _____
_____
Remarks (personal): _____
_____

Friday

Resting Pulse Rate	Weight At Rising

EXERCISE

Activity _____
_____
Time _____
Distance _____
Pace _____
Effort: ☐ Easy ☐ Moderate
         ☐ Hard ☐ Extreme

Remarks (fitness): _____
_____
Remarks (personal): _____
_____

Saturday

Resting Pulse Rate	Weight At Rising

EXERCISE

Activity _____
_____
Time _____
Distance _____
Pace _____
Effort: ☐ Easy ☐ Moderate
         ☐ Hard ☐ Extreme

Remarks (fitness): _____
_____
Remarks (personal): _____
_____

Sunday

Resting Pulse Rate	Weight At Rising

EXERCISE

Activity _____
_____
Time _____
Distance _____
Pace _____
Effort: ☐ Easy ☐ Moderate
         ☐ Hard ☐ Extreme

Remarks (fitness): _____
_____
Remarks (personal): _____
_____

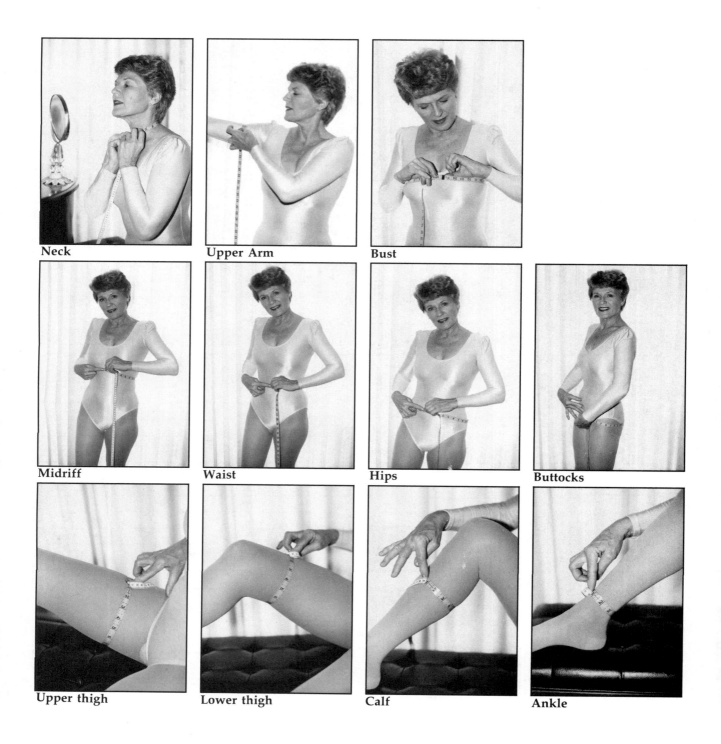

Neck

Upper Arm

Bust

Midriff

Waist

Hips

Buttocks

Upper thigh

Lower thigh

Calf

Ankle

Recording your monthly body measurements

In the empty boxes that correspond to the body part on the facing page, fill in your measurement at the end of this month. Don't be afraid to write the number large enough so that you can make quick reference to it from various months down the road. This will be a permanent record of your progress. Remember that better body sculpturing is a matter of inches, not pounds.

Neck

Upper Arm

Bust

Midriff

Waist

Hips

Buttocks

Upper thigh

Lower thigh

Calf

Ankle

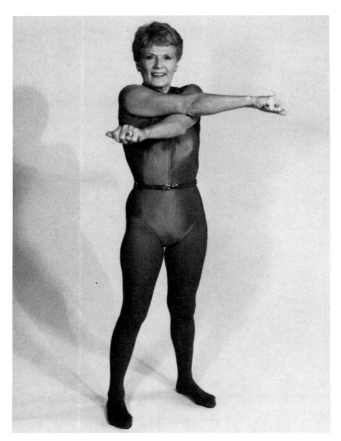

If God hadn't meant us to be fit, he wouldn't have given us the equipment to attain fitness. And the knowledge of how to use it.

Goals for this week:
1. _____
2. _____

Goals for this month:
1. _____
2. _____

Arm Crosses
Wonderful exercises for the upper back, shoulders and chest. Start from the same stance you used on the Arm Circles (on page 8). But instead of making circles, bring your arms across your chest, making a fist with hands, palms down. Then spread your arms back as far as possible, with head back, looking toward ceiling; returning to crossed position.

Apricot or Prune Whip
1½ cups apricot or prune pulp
1½ tbsp. lemon juice
⅓ cup honey
3 egg whites, stiffly beaten
chopped nuts

Mix pulp, lemon juice and honey: fold fruit mixture into egg whites. Serve with chopped nuts as a garnish. This mixture may also be piled into an oiled baking dish and baked at 275 degrees for 30-45 minutes.

Note: To make pulp, blend fresh or canned fruit in blender.

This week covers _____ , _____ , _____ , to _____ , _____ , _____ .
     month   day   year   month   day   year

Monday		E X E R C I S E	Activity _____ _____ Time _____ Distance _____ Pace _____ Effort: ☐ Easy ☐ Moderate ☐ Hard ☐ Extreme	Remarks (fitness): _____ _____ _____ Remarks (personal): _____ _____ _____
Resting Pulse Rate	Weight At Rising			
Tuesday		E X E R C I S E	Activity _____ _____ Time _____ Distance _____ Pace _____ Effort: ☐ Easy ☐ Moderate ☐ Hard ☐ Extreme	Remarks (fitness): _____ _____ _____ Remarks (personal): _____ _____ _____
Resting Pulse Rate	Weight At Rising			
Wednesday		E X E R C I S E	Activity _____ _____ Time _____ Distance _____ Pace _____ Effort: ☐ Easy ☐ Moderate ☐ Hard ☐ Extreme	Remarks (fitness): _____ _____ _____ Remarks (personal): _____ _____ _____
Resting Pulse Rate	Weight At Rising			
Thursday		E X E R C I S E	Activity _____ _____ Time _____ Distance _____ Pace _____ Effort: ☐ Easy ☐ Moderate ☐ Hard ☐ Extreme	Remarks (fitness): _____ _____ _____ Remarks (personal): _____ _____ _____
Resting Pulse Rate	Weight At Rising			
Friday		E X E R C I S E	Activity _____ _____ Time _____ Distance _____ Pace _____ Effort: ☐ Easy ☐ Moderate ☐ Hard ☐ Extreme	Remarks (fitness): _____ _____ _____ Remarks (personal): _____ _____ _____
Resting Pulse Rate	Weight At Rising			
Saturday		E X E R C I S E	Activity _____ _____ Time _____ Distance _____ Pace _____ Effort: ☐ Easy ☐ Moderate ☐ Hard ☐ Extreme	Remarks (fitness): _____ _____ _____ Remarks (personal): _____ _____ _____
Resting Pulse Rate	Weight At Rising			
Sunday		E X E R C I S E	Activity _____ _____ Time _____ Distance _____ Pace _____ Effort: ☐ Easy ☐ Moderate ☐ Hard ☐ Extreme	Remarks (fitness): _____ _____ _____ Remarks (personal): _____ _____ _____
Resting Pulse Rate	Weight At Rising			

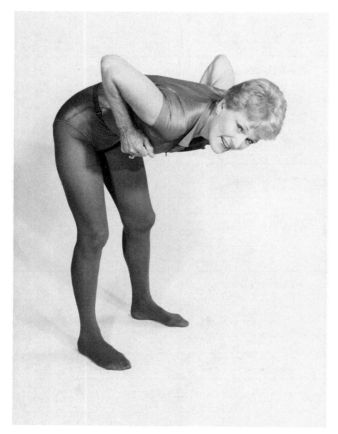

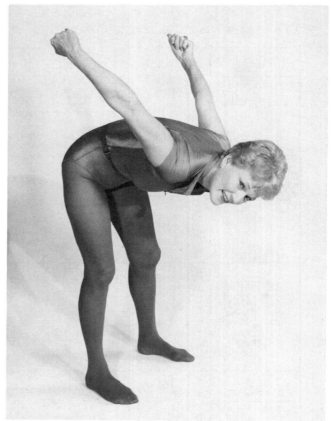

Arm Extensions

This exercise helps firm and tighten the backs of arms. Stand with your legs together or shoulder-width apart; bend over at waist, keeping elbows close to side and as high as possible. Then extend arms to the back with a smooth extension movement, trying to touch ceiling.

Goals for this week:

1. _____

2. _____

Goals for this month:

1. _____

2. _____

Elaine's Wheat Germ Muffins

¼ cup bran

1 cup raw wheat germ

⅔ cup milk

1 egg

¼ cup safflower oil

1 cup whole wheat flour (sifted)

2½ tsp. baking powder

¼ cup honey

½ cup raisins

Sift whole wheat flour, baking powder and salt together and then add other ingredients. Mix together. Bake in moderate oven (400 degrees) about 25 minutes.

The only good thing about cigarettes is that they eventually burn themselves out.

This week covers _____ , _____ , _____ , **to** _____ , _____ , _____ .
month   day   year   month   day   year

Monday	E X E R C I S E	Activity _____	Remarks (fitness): _____

Resting Pulse Rate	**Weight At Rising**

Time _____
Distance _____
Pace _____
Effort: ☐ Easy   ☐ Moderate
          ☐ Hard   ☐ Extreme

Remarks (personal): _____

Tuesday

| **Resting Pulse Rate** | **Weight At Rising** |

Activity _____
Time _____
Distance _____
Pace _____
Effort: ☐ Easy   ☐ Moderate
          ☐ Hard   ☐ Extreme

Remarks (fitness): _____
Remarks (personal): _____

Wednesday

| **Resting Pulse Rate** | **Weight At Rising** |

Activity _____
Time _____
Distance _____
Pace _____
Effort: ☐ Easy   ☐ Moderate
          ☐ Hard   ☐ Extreme

Remarks (fitness): _____
Remarks (personal): _____

Thursday

| **Resting Pulse Rate** | **Weight At Rising** |

Activity _____
Time _____
Distance _____
Pace _____
Effort: ☐ Easy   ☐ Moderate
          ☐ Hard   ☐ Extreme

Remarks (fitness): _____
Remarks (personal): _____

Friday

| **Resting Pulse Rate** | **Weight At Rising** |

Activity _____
Time _____
Distance _____
Pace _____
Effort: ☐ Easy   ☐ Moderate
          ☐ Hard   ☐ Extreme

Remarks (fitness): _____
Remarks (personal): _____

Saturday

| **Resting Pulse Rate** | **Weight At Rising** |

Activity _____
Time _____
Distance _____
Pace _____
Effort: ☐ Easy   ☐ Moderate
          ☐ Hard   ☐ Extreme

Remarks (fitness): _____
Remarks (personal): _____

Sunday

| **Resting Pulse Rate** | **Weight At Rising** |

Activity _____
Time _____
Distance _____
Pace _____
Effort: ☐ Easy   ☐ Moderate
          ☐ Hard   ☐ Extreme

Remarks (fitness): _____
Remarks (personal): _____

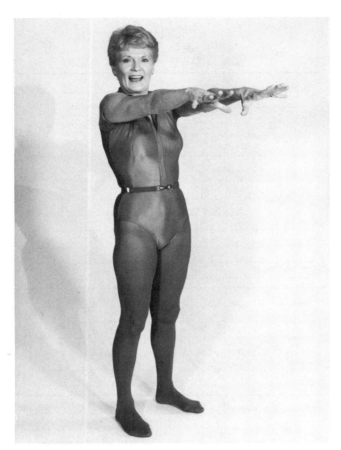
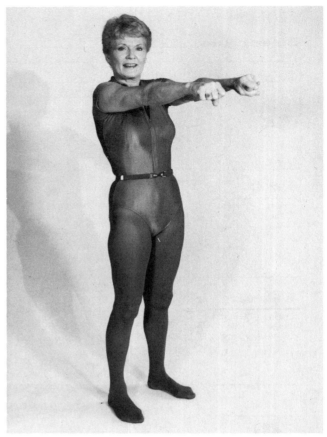

Hand Extension and Flex
Excellent exercise for strengthening hands, wrists and forearms. Stand with feet together or shoulder-width apart, arms out in front of you. Extend fingers to the maximum, then make a tight fist. Repeat until tired.

Elaine's Rice Dish

2 cups cooked brown rice
1 cup celery
1 cup bell pepper
1 cup chopped onion
1 cup mushrooms
garlic powder to taste
vegetable seasoning to taste

Lightly sauté celery, bell pepper, onions, and mushrooms. Add cooked rice. Season with garlic and your own seasonings to taste. Note: The secret of this recipe is not to overcook the vegetables. Keep them crisp!

Goals for this week:

1. _____

2. _____

Goals for this month:

1. _____

2. _____

The condition in which you keep your body reflects on what you feel about yourself, and you can't expect others to feel good about you if you don't.

16

This week covers _____ , _____ , _____ , to _____ , _____ , _____ .
month   day   year   month   day   year

Monday

Resting Pulse Rate	Weight At Rising

E X E R C I S E

Activity _____
_____
Time _____
Distance _____
Pace _____
Effort: ☐ Easy   ☐ Moderate
        ☐ Hard   ☐ Extreme

Remarks (fitness): _____
_____
_____

Remarks (personal): _____
_____
_____

Tuesday

Resting Pulse Rate	Weight At Rising

E X E R C I S E

Activity _____
_____
Time _____
Distance _____
Pace _____
Effort: ☐ Easy   ☐ Moderate
        ☐ Hard   ☐ Extreme

Remarks (fitness): _____
_____
_____

Remarks (personal): _____
_____
_____

Wednesday

Resting Pulse Rate	Weight At Rising

E X E R C I S E

Activity _____
_____
Time _____
Distance _____
Pace _____
Effort: ☐ Easy   ☐ Moderate
        ☐ Hard   ☐ Extreme

Remarks (fitness): _____
_____
_____

Remarks (personal): _____
_____
_____

Thursday

Resting Pulse Rate	Weight At Rising

E X E R C I S E

Activity _____
_____
Time _____
Distance _____
Pace _____
Effort: ☐ Easy   ☐ Moderate
        ☐ Hard   ☐ Extreme

Remarks (fitness): _____
_____
_____

Remarks (personal): _____
_____
_____

Friday

Resting Pulse Rate	Weight At Rising

E X E R C I S E

Activity _____
_____
Time _____
Distance _____
Pace _____
Effort: ☐ Easy   ☐ Moderate
        ☐ Hard   ☐ Extreme

Remarks (fitness): _____
_____
_____

Remarks (personal): _____
_____
_____

Saturday

Resting Pulse Rate	Weight At Rising

E X E R C I S E

Activity _____
_____
Time _____
Distance _____
Pace _____
Effort: ☐ Easy   ☐ Moderate
        ☐ Hard   ☐ Extreme

Remarks (fitness): _____
_____
_____

Remarks (personal): _____
_____
_____

Sunday

Resting Pulse Rate	Weight At Rising

E X E R C I S E

Activity _____
_____
Time _____
Distance _____
Pace _____
Effort: ☐ Easy   ☐ Moderate
        ☐ Hard   ☐ Extreme

Remarks (fitness): _____
_____
_____

Remarks (personal): _____
_____
_____

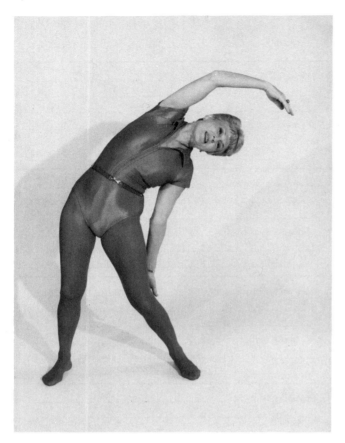

Side Bends
The basic side bend is an excellent way of keeping the sides of your waist supple and toned. Stand with your feet shoulder-width apart, right hand behind head, left hand hanging like you have a weight in it. Bend to the left and then bend to the right. Alternate. Repeat with left hand behind head.

One nice thing about taking a walk to the store instead of taking the car is that you never lock your keys inside yourself by mistake.

Goals for this week:
1. _____
2. _____
Goals for this month:
1. _____
2. _____

Sweet Potatoes and Apples
4 medium size sweet potatoes
4 medium size apples
½ to ¾ cup honey
½ tsp. cinnamon
1 tsp. lemon juice
2 tbsp. safflower oil
½ cup warm water

Cook potatoes until tender; cool, peel and cut into 1-inch-thick slices. Core apples and slice into ½-inch rings. Arrange potatoes and apples in alternate layers in oiled baking dish. Mix together honey, cinnamon, oil and sprinkle part of this mixture and lemon juice over each layer. Add water, cover and bake at 375 degrees for 35 minutes. Remove cover and bake another 10 minutes. Serves 6.

This week covers _____ , _____ , _____ , to _____ , _____ , _____ .
  month   day   year   month   day   year

Monday

Resting Pulse Rate	Weight At Rising

EXERCISE

Activity _____
_____
Time _____
Distance _____
Pace _____
Effort: ☐ Easy   ☐ Moderate
         ☐ Hard   ☐ Extreme

Remarks (fitness): _____
_____
Remarks (personal): _____
_____
_____

Tuesday

Resting Pulse Rate	Weight At Rising

EXERCISE

Activity _____
_____
Time _____
Distance _____
Pace _____
Effort: ☐ Easy   ☐ Moderate
         ☐ Hard   ☐ Extreme

Remarks (fitness): _____
_____
Remarks (personal): _____
_____
_____

Wednesday

Resting Pulse Rate	Weight At Rising

EXERCISE

Activity _____
_____
Time _____
Distance _____
Pace _____
Effort: ☐ Easy   ☐ Moderate
         ☐ Hard   ☐ Extreme

Remarks (fitness): _____
_____
Remarks (personal): _____
_____
_____

Thursday

Resting Pulse Rate	Weight At Rising

EXERCISE

Activity _____
_____
Time _____
Distance _____
Pace _____
Effort: ☐ Easy   ☐ Moderate
         ☐ Hard   ☐ Extreme

Remarks (fitness): _____
_____
Remarks (personal): _____
_____
_____

Friday

Resting Pulse Rate	Weight At Rising

EXERCISE

Activity _____
_____
Time _____
Distance _____
Pace _____
Effort: ☐ Easy   ☐ Moderate
         ☐ Hard   ☐ Extreme

Remarks (fitness): _____
_____
Remarks (personal): _____
_____
_____

Saturday

Resting Pulse Rate	Weight At Rising

EXERCISE

Activity _____
_____
Time _____
Distance _____
Pace _____
Effort: ☐ Easy   ☐ Moderate
         ☐ Hard   ☐ Extreme

Remarks (fitness): _____
_____
Remarks (personal): _____
_____
_____

Sunday

Resting Pulse Rate	Weight At Rising

EXERCISE

Activity _____
_____
Time _____
Distance _____
Pace _____
Effort: ☐ Easy   ☐ Moderate
         ☐ Hard   ☐ Extreme

Remarks (fitness): _____
_____
Remarks (personal): _____
_____
_____

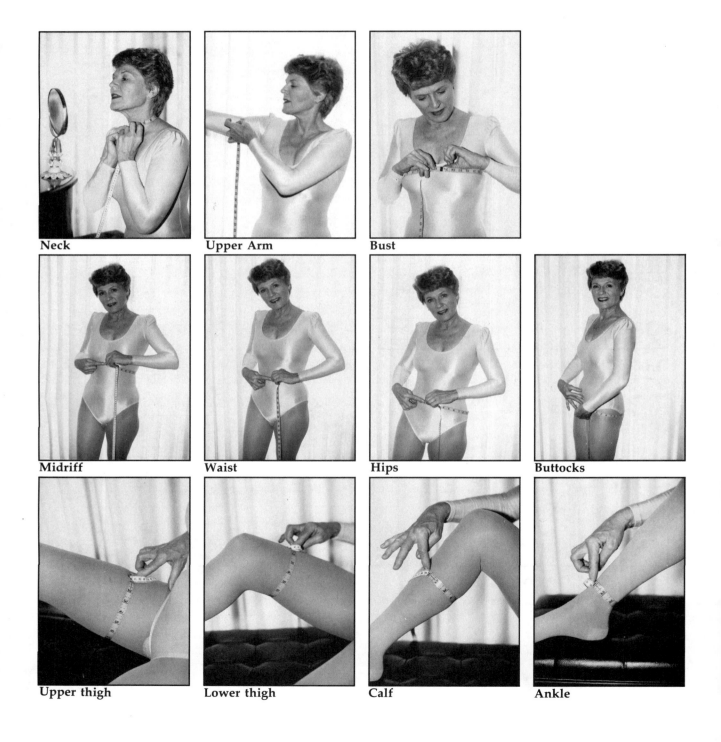

Neck

Upper Arm

Bust

Midriff

Waist

Hips

Buttocks

Upper thigh

Lower thigh

Calf

Ankle

Neck

Upper Arm

Bust

Midriff

Waist

Hips

Buttocks

Upper thigh

Lower thigh

Calf

Ankle

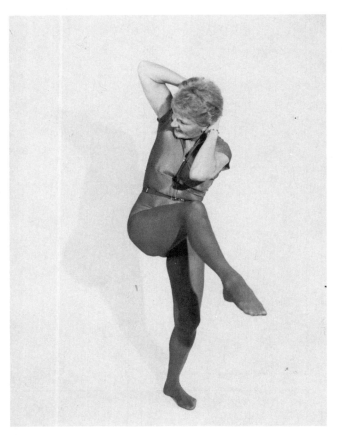

One good meal a day will give you better nourishment than a half-dozen inferior meals. (And it'll cost you less, pile on less calories, and will keep you feeling light enough to keep fit.) So if one good meal a day is good, two must be better.

Knee into Chest (*standing*)
Excellent waist trimmer. Stand erect with your legs shoulder-width apart; with hands behind head, bring right knee up and try to touch left elbow. Make sure that you bring knee up to the elbow, not elbow down to the knee.

Goals for this week:

1. _____

2. _____

Goals for this month:

1. _____

2. _____

Elaine's Chicken Wings

6 chicken wings
2 tbsp. safflower oil
1 tbsp. soy sauce
garlic powder and seasonings to taste
natural brown rice (long or short grain); use package instructions

Mix ingredients for sauce. Let chicken wings marinate for a while in the sauce. (If you're in a hurry, just dip on both sides.) Broil wings to desired brownness and doneness. Serve chicken wings over brown rice. *Variation:* Bake wings for approximately 30 minutes in 350 degree oven.

This week covers _____ , _____ , _____ , to _____ , _____ , _____ .
month   day   year   month   day   year

Monday

Resting Pulse Rate	Weight At Rising

EXERCISE

Activity _____
_____
Time _____
Distance _____
Pace _____
Effort:　□ Easy　　□ Moderate
　　　　□ Hard　　□ Extreme

Remarks (fitness): _____
_____
Remarks (personal): _____
_____

Tuesday

Resting Pulse Rate	Weight At Rising

EXERCISE

Activity _____
_____
Time _____
Distance _____
Pace _____
Effort:　□ Easy　　□ Moderate
　　　　□ Hard　　□ Extreme

Remarks (fitness): _____
_____
Remarks (personal): _____
_____

Wednesday

Resting Pulse Rate	Weight At Rising

EXERCISE

Activity _____
_____
Time _____
Distance _____
Pace _____
Effort:　□ Easy　　□ Moderate
　　　　□ Hard　　□ Extreme

Remarks (fitness): _____
_____
Remarks (personal): _____
_____

Thursday

Resting Pulse Rate	Weight At Rising

EXERCISE

Activity _____
_____
Time _____
Distance _____
Pace _____
Effort:　□ Easy　　□ Moderate
　　　　□ Hard　　□ Extreme

Remarks (fitness): _____
_____
Remarks (personal): _____
_____

Friday

Resting Pulse Rate	Weight At Rising

EXERCISE

Activity _____
_____
Time _____
Distance _____
Pace _____
Effort:　□ Easy　　□ Moderate
　　　　□ Hard　　□ Extreme

Remarks (fitness): _____
_____
Remarks (personal): _____
_____

Saturday

Resting Pulse Rate	Weight At Rising

EXERCISE

Activity _____
_____
Time _____
Distance _____
Pace _____
Effort:　□ Easy　　□ Moderate
　　　　□ Hard　　□ Extreme

Remarks (fitness): _____
_____
Remarks (personal): _____
_____

Sunday

Resting Pulse Rate	Weight At Rising

EXERCISE

Activity _____
_____
Time _____
Distance _____
Pace _____
Effort:　□ Easy　　□ Moderate
　　　　□ Hard　　□ Extreme

Remarks (fitness): _____
_____
Remarks (personal): _____
_____

There is really no short-cut to fitness; but when you're fit, your fitness won't short-change you.

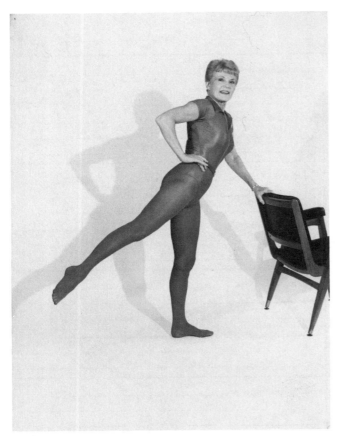

Standing Leg Extensions
The leg extension to the back works the muscles in the lower back, buttocks and back of leg. Stand erect with feet shoulder-width apart, hands on hips or one hand on a chair to help keep your balance. Extend your right leg to the back as far as possible in a smooth motion.

Goals for this week:
1. _____
2. _____

Goals for this month:
1. _____
2. _____

Cottage Cheese Pie
1 envelope unflavored gelatin
¼ cup cold water
¼ cup hot water
1 tsp. grated lemon rind
1 tbsp. honey
1 cup unsweetened pineapple juice
1 cup low-fat cottage cheese
   whipped in blender
freshly grated coconut

Soften gelatin in cold water. Add hot water and stir to dissolve. Add the remaining ingredients, except coconut. Lightly oil 9-inch pie plate and press coconut to form shell. Pour filling in (over large spoon) so as not to separate coconut. Chill until set.

This week covers _____ , _____ , _____ , to _____ , _____ , _____ .
month   day   year   month   day   year

Monday	E	Activity _____	Remarks (fitness): _____
	X	_____	_____
Resting Pulse Rate / **Weight At Rising**	E R C I S E	Time _____ Distance _____ Pace _____ Effort: ☐ Easy ☐ Moderate ☐ Hard ☐ Extreme	Remarks (personal): _____ _____ _____

Tuesday	E	Activity _____	Remarks (fitness): _____
	X	_____	_____
Resting Pulse Rate / **Weight At Rising**	E R C I S E	Time _____ Distance _____ Pace _____ Effort: ☐ Easy ☐ Moderate ☐ Hard ☐ Extreme	Remarks (personal): _____ _____ _____

Wednesday	E	Activity _____	Remarks (fitness): _____
	X	_____	_____
Resting Pulse Rate / **Weight At Rising**	E R C I S E	Time _____ Distance _____ Pace _____ Effort: ☐ Easy ☐ Moderate ☐ Hard ☐ Extreme	Remarks (personal): _____ _____ _____

Thursday	E	Activity _____	Remarks (fitness): _____
	X	_____	_____
Resting Pulse Rate / **Weight At Rising**	E R C I S E	Time _____ Distance _____ Pace _____ Effort: ☐ Easy ☐ Moderate ☐ Hard ☐ Extreme	Remarks (personal): _____ _____ _____

Friday	E	Activity _____	Remarks (fitness): _____
	X	_____	_____
Resting Pulse Rate / **Weight At Rising**	E R C I S E	Time _____ Distance _____ Pace _____ Effort: ☐ Easy ☐ Moderate ☐ Hard ☐ Extreme	Remarks (personal): _____ _____ _____

Saturday	E	Activity _____	Remarks (fitness): _____
	X	_____	_____
Resting Pulse Rate / **Weight At Rising**	E R C I S E	Time _____ Distance _____ Pace _____ Effort: ☐ Easy ☐ Moderate ☐ Hard ☐ Extreme	Remarks (personal): _____ _____ _____

Sunday	E	Activity _____	Remarks (fitness): _____
	X	_____	_____
Resting Pulse Rate / **Weight At Rising**	E R C I S E	Time _____ Distance _____ Pace _____ Effort: ☐ Easy ☐ Moderate ☐ Hard ☐ Extreme	Remarks (personal): _____ _____ _____

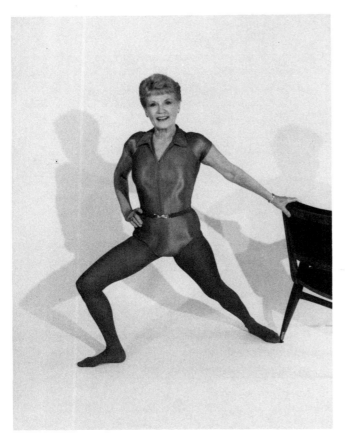

You'd be surprised how quickly you can turn a gloomy day into a bright one by getting your blood rushing by a good workout.

Goals for this week:
1. _____
2. _____

Goals for this month:
1. _____
2. _____

Leg Lunges to the Side
I believe that this is one of the best exercises for the hips and thighs. Stand erect, hands on hips, or hold on to a chair to keep your balance. Lunge to the right with right leg...step back and lunge to the left on opposite leg.

Broiled Oranges and Grapes
**2 large oranges
1 cup Thompson grapes, halved
2 tbsp. safflower oil
2 tbsp. honey
¼ tsp. cinnamon
flaked coconut**

Halve oranges in a saw-toothed cut. Remove fruit, discard membrane. Combine oranges, grapes, oil, honey and cinnamon. Spoon into orange skins. Place in shallow baking pan and sprinkle with coconut. Broil 5-6 inches under broiler about 2-3 minutes or until heated—or until coconut is brown.

This week covers _____ , _____ , _____ , to _____ , _____ , _____ .
                     month   day   year   month   day   year

Monday

Resting Pulse Rate	Weight At Rising

EXERCISE

Activity _____
_____
Time _____
Distance _____
Pace _____
Effort: ☐ Easy ☐ Moderate
       ☐ Hard ☐ Extreme

Remarks (fitness): _____
_____
Remarks (personal): _____
_____

Tuesday

Resting Pulse Rate	Weight At Rising

EXERCISE

Activity _____
_____
Time _____
Distance _____
Pace _____
Effort: ☐ Easy ☐ Moderate
       ☐ Hard ☐ Extreme

Remarks (fitness): _____
_____
Remarks (personal): _____
_____

Wednesday

Resting Pulse Rate	Weight At Rising

EXERCISE

Activity _____
_____
Time _____
Distance _____
Pace _____
Effort: ☐ Easy ☐ Moderate
       ☐ Hard ☐ Extreme

Remarks (fitness): _____
_____
Remarks (personal): _____
_____

Thursday

Resting Pulse Rate	Weight At Rising

EXERCISE

Activity _____
_____
Time _____
Distance _____
Pace _____
Effort: ☐ Easy ☐ Moderate
       ☐ Hard ☐ Extreme

Remarks (fitness): _____
_____
Remarks (personal): _____
_____

Friday

Resting Pulse Rate	Weight At Rising

EXERCISE

Activity _____
_____
Time _____
Distance _____
Pace _____
Effort: ☐ Easy ☐ Moderate
       ☐ Hard ☐ Extreme

Remarks (fitness): _____
_____
Remarks (personal): _____
_____

Saturday

Resting Pulse Rate	Weight At Rising

EXERCISE

Activity _____
_____
Time _____
Distance _____
Pace _____
Effort: ☐ Easy ☐ Moderate
       ☐ Hard ☐ Extreme

Remarks (fitness): _____
_____
Remarks (personal): _____
_____

Sunday

Resting Pulse Rate	Weight At Rising

EXERCISE

Activity _____
_____
Time _____
Distance _____
Pace _____
Effort: ☐ Easy ☐ Moderate
       ☐ Hard ☐ Extreme

Remarks (fitness): _____
_____
Remarks (personal): _____
_____

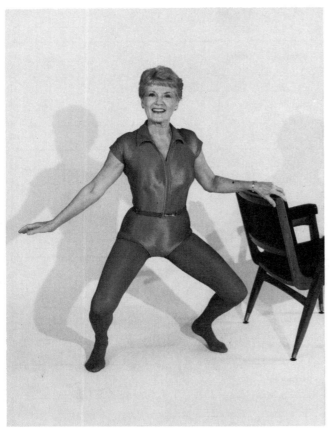

Half Squats
Very effective for the front of your thighs.
Half squats are very helpful for those of you
who cannot do "deep" knee bends. Stand
erect, feet shoulder-width apart, bend your
knees, lean back slightly trying to keep your
shoulders behind your heels. Bend and
straighten 5 times; increasing as you get
stronger. *Variation:* Walk forward and backward
in this position. You should feel the muscles
working in the front of your thighs.

It is nice to exercise with
other people, but never
blame other people for your
being unable to exercise;
depend on yourself to
motivate yourself, and on
your friends to celebrate the
feat with you.

Goals for this week:
1. _____
2. _____

Goals for this month:
1. _____
2. _____

Low Sodium Dressing
(From American Lupus Society)

¾ cup rice vinegar
¼ cup sesame oil
½ tbsp. powdered ginger
fresh garlic juice or dash garlic
    powder
few drops Angostura bitters
¼ tsp. basil
2 tbsp. chopped parsley
1 California laurel bay leaf
¼ tbsp. dried mustard

Make a paste of all ingredients before
adding rice vinegar. Mix well and serve.

This week covers _____ , _____ , _____ , to _____ , _____ , _____ .
month　　　　　day　　　　　year　　　　　　month　　　　　day　　　　　year

Monday	E	Activity _____	Remarks (fitness): _____
Resting Pulse Rate / **Weight At Rising**	X E R C I S E	_____ Time _____ Distance _____ Pace _____ Effort: ☐ Easy　☐ Moderate ☐ Hard　☐ Extreme	_____ Remarks (personal): _____ _____

Tuesday	E	Activity _____	Remarks (fitness): _____
Resting Pulse Rate / **Weight At Rising**	X E R C I S E	_____ Time _____ Distance _____ Pace _____ Effort: ☐ Easy　☐ Moderate ☐ Hard　☐ Extreme	_____ Remarks (personal): _____ _____

Wednesday	E	Activity _____	Remarks (fitness): _____
Resting Pulse Rate / **Weight At Rising**	X E R C I S E	_____ Time _____ Distance _____ Pace _____ Effort: ☐ Easy　☐ Moderate ☐ Hard　☐ Extreme	_____ Remarks (personal): _____ _____

Thursday	E	Activity _____	Remarks (fitness): _____
Resting Pulse Rate / **Weight At Rising**	X E R C I S E	_____ Time _____ Distance _____ Pace _____ Effort: ☐ Easy　☐ Moderate ☐ Hard　☐ Extreme	_____ Remarks (personal): _____ _____

Friday	E	Activity _____	Remarks (fitness): _____
Resting Pulse Rate / **Weight At Rising**	X E R C I S E	_____ Time _____ Distance _____ Pace _____ Effort: ☐ Easy　☐ Moderate ☐ Hard　☐ Extreme	_____ Remarks (personal): _____ _____

Saturday	E	Activity _____	Remarks (fitness): _____
Resting Pulse Rate / **Weight At Rising**	X E R C I S E	_____ Time _____ Distance _____ Pace _____ Effort: ☐ Easy　☐ Moderate ☐ Hard　☐ Extreme	_____ Remarks (personal): _____ _____

Sunday	E	Activity _____	Remarks (fitness): _____
Resting Pulse Rate / **Weight At Rising**	X E R C I S E	_____ Time _____ Distance _____ Pace _____ Effort: ☐ Easy　☐ Moderate ☐ Hard　☐ Extreme	_____ Remarks (personal): _____ _____

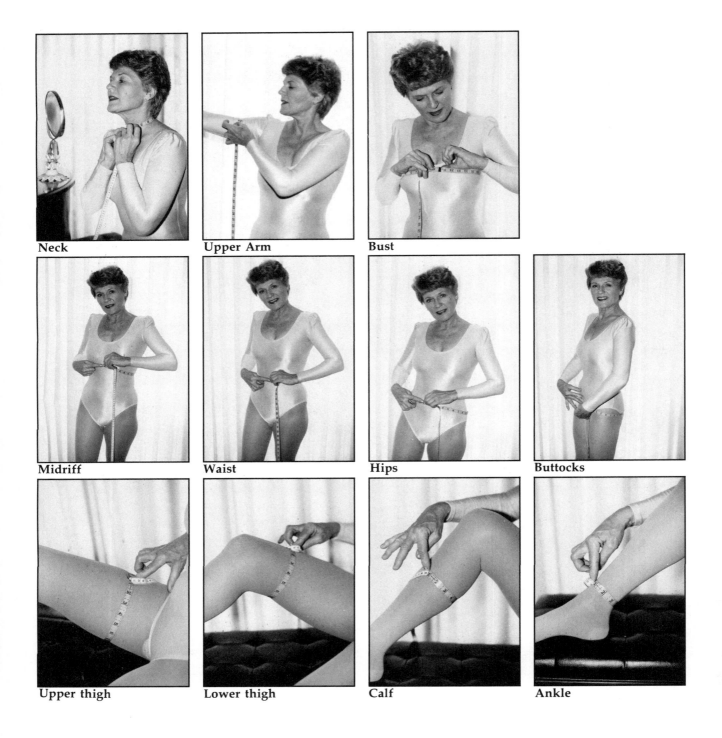

Neck

Upper Arm

Bust

Midriff

Waist

Hips

Buttocks

Upper thigh

Lower thigh

Calf

Ankle

Neck

Upper Arm

Bust

Midriff

Waist

Hips

Buttocks

Upper thigh

Lower thigh

Calf

Ankle

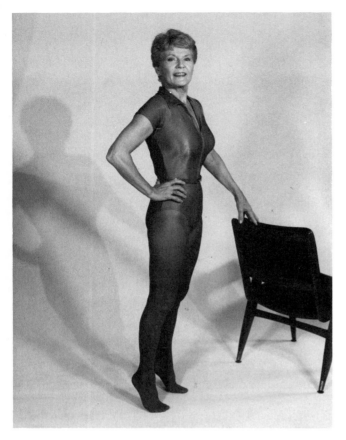

**Thinking good thoughts
makes you feel good;
feeling good gives you
a jump on making your
life better.**

Goals for this week:
1. _____
2. _____

Goals for this month:
1. _____
2. _____

Toe Raises

Toe raises are a strengthening and flexibility exercise for the back and lower legs. Stand erect, with your feet in a comfortable position. Raise yourself up on your toes, for a count of two, and then lower yourself back to starting position. Repeat 10 to 25 times. Great for the calf of the leg. *Variation:* Repeat same exercise with toes pointed in and toes pointed out.

Fruit Salad

3 lettuce leaves, torn
1 medium apple, with peel, diced
6 grapes (red, green or black)
**raisins, sunflower seeds, nuts
(optional)**
**dressing: 1 cup yogurt, thinned with
2 tbsp. fruit juice (concentrate)**

Place lettuce in plate, arrange apple and grapes. Top with dressing and sprinkle with raisins, sunflower seeds, nuts, etc.

This week covers _____ , _____ , _____ , to _____ , _____ , _____ .

month   day   year   month   day   year

Monday

Resting Pulse Rate	Weight At Rising

E X E R C I S E

Activity _____
_____
Time _____
Distance _____
Pace _____
Effort: ☐ Easy ☐ Moderate
       ☐ Hard ☐ Extreme

Remarks (fitness): _____
_____
Remarks (personal): _____
_____

Tuesday

Resting Pulse Rate	Weight At Rising

E X E R C I S E

Activity _____
_____
Time _____
Distance _____
Pace _____
Effort: ☐ Easy ☐ Moderate
       ☐ Hard ☐ Extreme

Remarks (fitness): _____
_____
Remarks (personal): _____
_____

Wednesday

Resting Pulse Rate	Weight At Rising

E X E R C I S E

Activity _____
_____
Time _____
Distance _____
Pace _____
Effort: ☐ Easy ☐ Moderate
       ☐ Hard ☐ Extreme

Remarks (fitness): _____
_____
Remarks (personal): _____
_____

Thursday

Resting Pulse Rate	Weight At Rising

E X E R C I S E

Activity _____
_____
Time _____
Distance _____
Pace _____
Effort: ☐ Easy ☐ Moderate
       ☐ Hard ☐ Extreme

Remarks (fitness): _____
_____
Remarks (personal): _____
_____

Friday

Resting Pulse Rate	Weight At Rising

E X E R C I S E

Activity _____
_____
Time _____
Distance _____
Pace _____
Effort: ☐ Easy ☐ Moderate
       ☐ Hard ☐ Extreme

Remarks (fitness): _____
_____
Remarks (personal): _____
_____

Saturday

Resting Pulse Rate	Weight At Rising

E X E R C I S E

Activity _____
_____
Time _____
Distance _____
Pace _____
Effort: ☐ Easy ☐ Moderate
       ☐ Hard ☐ Extreme

Remarks (fitness): _____
_____
Remarks (personal): _____
_____

Sunday

Resting Pulse Rate	Weight At Rising

E X E R C I S E

Activity _____
Time _____
Distance _____
Pace _____
Effort: ☐ Easy ☐ Moderate
       ☐ Hard ☐ Extreme

Remarks (fitness): _____
_____
Remarks (personal): _____
_____

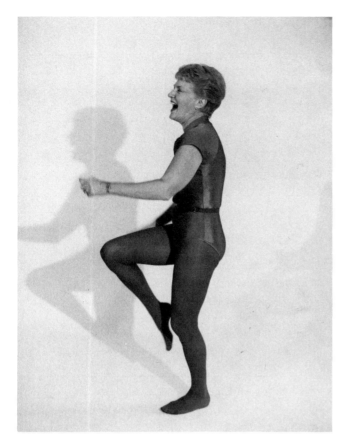

Fitness has a way of building upon itself. Once you get fit, it becomes easy to build upon your foundation.

Goals for this week:

1. _____

2. _____

Goals for this month:

1. _____

2. _____

Running in Place

Everyone knows how to run in place. Great aerobic/cardiovascular exercise. Start out by easy jogging and work up to bringing your knees higher each day. Keep knees pulled in toward chest. The higher your knees come up, the more difficult the exercise. Increase a little more each day.

White Radish and Jicama Salad

1 cup grated white radish
¼ cup grated carrot
¼ cup grated jicama
1 cucumber

Arrange grated vegetables on lettuce leaves in layers. Slice cucumber with peel and arrange around plate. Top with favorite dressing. For fancy slices, score cucumber.

This week covers _____ , _____ , _____ , to _____ , _____ , _____ .
month   day   year   month   day   year

Monday

Resting Pulse Rate	Weight At Rising

EXERCISE

Activity _____
_____
Time _____
Distance _____
Pace _____
Effort: ☐ Easy ☐ Moderate
☐ Hard ☐ Extreme

Remarks (fitness): _____
_____
Remarks (personal): _____
_____

Tuesday

Resting Pulse Rate	Weight At Rising

EXERCISE

Activity _____
_____
Time _____
Distance _____
Pace _____
Effort: ☐ Easy ☐ Moderate
☐ Hard ☐ Extreme

Remarks (fitness): _____
_____
Remarks (personal): _____
_____

Wednesday

Resting Pulse Rate	Weight At Rising

EXERCISE

Activity _____
_____
Time _____
Distance _____
Pace _____
Effort: ☐ Easy ☐ Moderate
☐ Hard ☐ Extreme

Remarks (fitness): _____
_____
Remarks (personal): _____
_____

Thursday

Resting Pulse Rate	Weight At Rising

EXERCISE

Activity _____
_____
Time _____
Distance _____
Pace _____
Effort: ☐ Easy ☐ Moderate
☐ Hard ☐ Extreme

Remarks (fitness): _____
_____
Remarks (personal): _____
_____

Friday

Resting Pulse Rate	Weight At Rising

EXERCISE

Activity _____
_____
Time _____
Distance _____
Pace _____
Effort: ☐ Easy ☐ Moderate
☐ Hard ☐ Extreme

Remarks (fitness): _____
_____
Remarks (personal): _____
_____

Saturday

Resting Pulse Rate	Weight At Rising

EXERCISE

Activity _____
_____
Time _____
Distance _____
Pace _____
Effort: ☐ Easy ☐ Moderate
☐ Hard ☐ Extreme

Remarks (fitness): _____
_____
Remarks (personal): _____
_____

Sunday

Resting Pulse Rate	Weight At Rising

EXERCISE

Activity _____
_____
Time _____
Distance _____
Pace _____
Effort: ☐ Easy ☐ Moderate
☐ Hard ☐ Extreme

Remarks (fitness): _____
_____
Remarks (personal): _____
_____

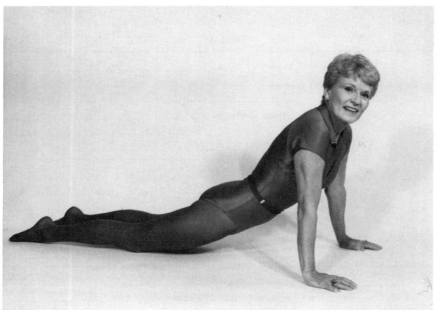

Push-Ups

One of the age-old stand-bys of exercising is the "push-up." Push-ups are excellent for building up the back of arms, shoulders and chest. Notice that I stay on my knees and thighs, rather than coming up on my toes. This cuts down on the weight you have to lift. Do this one as many times as is comfortable.

Goals for this week:

1. _____

2. _____

Goals for this month:

1. _____

2. _____

The best way to prevent yourself from getting fit is to tell yourself you can't get fit; luckily, the reverse strategy also works.

Glazed Chicken with Mustard Sauce

6 chicken legs with thighs
slivered almonds

Place 6 legs with thighs in greased baking dish. Cover with mustard sauce (recipe below) and bake at 400 degrees for half an hour. Sprinkle with slivered almonds and leave in oven with temperature off for another 10 minutes. During the initial baking, you may baste periodically.

Mustard Sauce for Chicken

½ cup honey
½ cup Grey Poupon Dijon mustard
1 tsp. lemon juice
1 tsp. onion
½ tsp. curry powder

Mix ingredients in small bowl until thoroughly mixed together.

This week covers _____ , _____ , _____ , to _____ , _____ , _____ .
month   day   year   month   day   year

Monday

Resting Pulse Rate	Weight At Rising

E X E R C I S E

Activity _____
_____
Time _____
Distance _____
Pace _____
Effort: ☐ Easy ☐ Moderate ☐ Hard ☐ Extreme

Remarks (fitness): _____
_____

Remarks (personal): _____
_____

Tuesday

Resting Pulse Rate	Weight At Rising

E X E R C I S E

Activity _____
_____
Time _____
Distance _____
Pace _____
Effort: ☐ Easy ☐ Moderate ☐ Hard ☐ Extreme

Remarks (fitness): _____
_____

Remarks (personal): _____
_____

Wednesday

Resting Pulse Rate	Weight At Rising

E X E R C I S E

Activity _____
_____
Time _____
Distance _____
Pace _____
Effort: ☐ Easy ☐ Moderate ☐ Hard ☐ Extreme

Remarks (fitness): _____
_____

Remarks (personal): _____
_____

Thursday

Resting Pulse Rate	Weight At Rising

E X E R C I S E

Activity _____
_____
Time _____
Distance _____
Pace _____
Effort: ☐ Easy ☐ Moderate ☐ Hard ☐ Extreme

Remarks (fitness): _____
_____

Remarks (personal): _____
_____

Friday

Resting Pulse Rate	Weight At Rising

E X E R C I S E

Activity _____
_____
Time _____
Distance _____
Pace _____
Effort: ☐ Easy ☐ Moderate ☐ Hard ☐ Extreme

Remarks (fitness): _____
_____

Remarks (personal): _____
_____

Saturday

Resting Pulse Rate	Weight At Rising

E X E R C I S E

Activity _____
_____
Time _____
Distance _____
Pace _____
Effort: ☐ Easy ☐ Moderate ☐ Hard ☐ Extreme

Remarks (fitness): _____
_____

Remarks (personal): _____
_____

Sunday

Resting Pulse Rate	Weight At Rising

E X E R C I S E

Activity _____
_____
Time _____
Distance _____
Pace _____
Effort: ☐ Easy ☐ Moderate ☐ Hard ☐ Extreme

Remarks (fitness): _____
_____

Remarks (personal): _____
_____

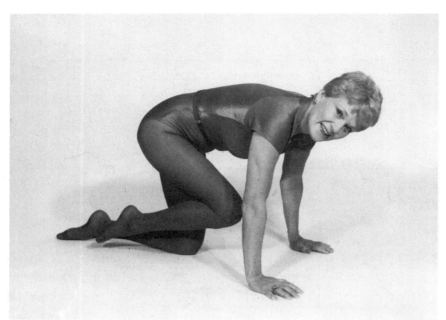

Knee into Chest
Sometimes called "donkey kicks;" only do not kick into the exercise. It is important to remember that you never kick, you lift your leg. On hands and knees, round back, head down, try to touch your knee to your nose. From this position, extend your leg to the back, arching your back and looking toward ceiling. This exercise is great for your waist, stomach, lower back and posture; everything from the back of the head to the bottom of the foot.

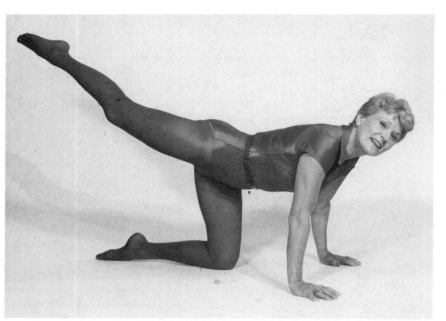

Get fit. Think fit.
Be fit. Stay fit.

Goals for this week:
1. _____
2. _____

Goals for this month:
1. _____
2. _____

Banana Toast
½ to 1 whole banana
1 egg
1 slice whole grain bread
season to taste with nutmeg, cinnamon

Put banana in blender or mash. Add egg and spices. Mix well. Dip slice of bread in mixture and brown slightly on each side in non-stick pan. Similar to French toast.

This week covers _____ , _____ , _____ , **to** _____ , _____ , _____ .
month   day   year   month   day   year

Monday

Resting Pulse Rate	Weight At Rising

E X E R C I S E

Activity _____
_____
Time _____
Distance _____
Pace _____
Effort: ☐ Easy ☐ Moderate
☐ Hard ☐ Extreme

Remarks (fitness): _____
_____
_____
Remarks (personal): _____
_____
_____

Tuesday

Resting Pulse Rate	Weight At Rising

E X E R C I S E

Activity _____
_____
Time _____
Distance _____
Pace _____
Effort: ☐ Easy ☐ Moderate
☐ Hard ☐ Extreme

Remarks (fitness): _____
_____
_____
Remarks (personal): _____
_____
_____

Wednesday

Resting Pulse Rate	Weight At Rising

E X E R C I S E

Activity _____
_____
Time _____
Distance _____
Pace _____
Effort: ☐ Easy ☐ Moderate
☐ Hard ☐ Extreme

Remarks (fitness): _____
_____
_____
Remarks (personal): _____
_____
_____

Thursday

Resting Pulse Rate	Weight At Rising

E X E R C I S E

Activity _____
_____
Time _____
Distance _____
Pace _____
Effort: ☐ Easy ☐ Moderate
☐ Hard ☐ Extreme

Remarks (fitness): _____
_____
_____
Remarks (personal): _____
_____
_____

Friday

Resting Pulse Rate	Weight At Rising

E X E R C I S E

Activity _____
_____
Time _____
Distance _____
Pace _____
Effort: ☐ Easy ☐ Moderate
☐ Hard ☐ Extreme

Remarks (fitness): _____
_____
_____
Remarks (personal): _____
_____
_____

Saturday

Resting Pulse Rate	Weight At Rising

E X E R C I S E

Activity _____
_____
Time _____
Distance _____
Pace _____
Effort: ☐ Easy ☐ Moderate
☐ Hard ☐ Extreme

Remarks (fitness): _____
_____
_____
Remarks (personal): _____
_____
_____

Sunday

Resting Pulse Rate	Weight At Rising

E X E R C I S E

Activity _____
_____
Time _____
Distance _____
Pace _____
Effort: ☐ Easy ☐ Moderate
☐ Hard ☐ Extreme

Remarks (fitness): _____
_____
_____
Remarks (personal): _____
_____
_____

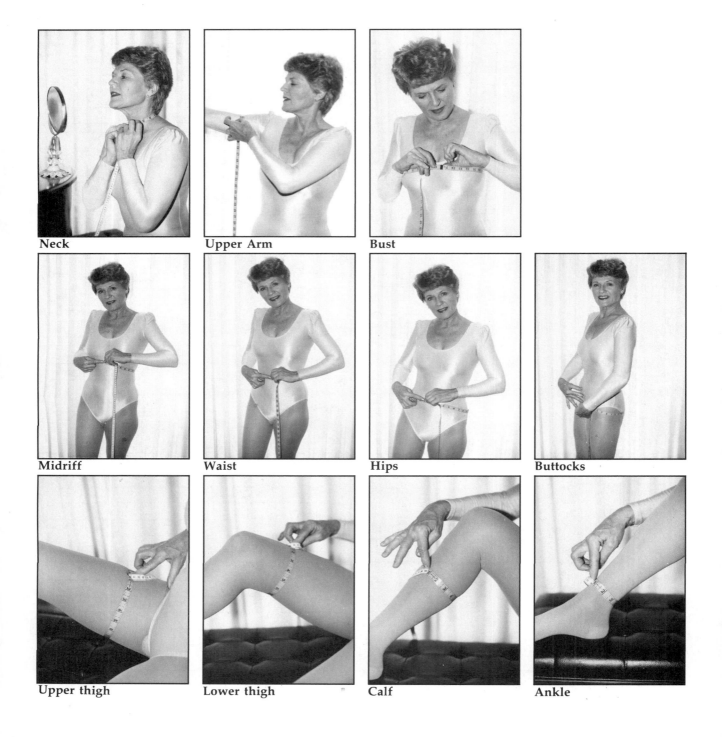

Neck

Upper Arm

Bust

Midriff

Waist

Hips

Buttocks

Upper thigh

Lower thigh

Calf

Ankle

Neck

Upper Arm

Bust

Midriff

Waist

Hips

Buttocks

Upper thigh

Lower thigh

Calf

Ankle

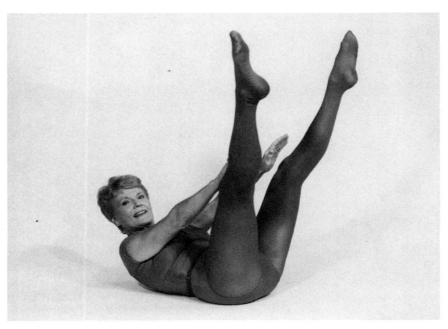

Sit-Ups to Feet
This exercise helps to tone and firm your midsection. Lie on your back, hands above head, with legs approximately two feet apart. Now, in one smooth motion, pull yourself up, bringing your hands between your knees. Don't worry if you cannot get up all the way; you are still getting benefit from the exercise. Do as many as you can. Make haste slowly. Do not overdo. *Variation:* put feet against wall.

Goals for this week:
1. _____
2. _____

Goals for this month:
1. _____
2. _____

A person will get fit only when that person is ready. So missionary work on behalf of fitness is folly. But good example isn't.

Shrimp/Avocado/Papaya Salad
½ avocado
½ papaya
scoop of baby shrimp

On bed of lettuce, place the mound of baby shrimp; slice ½ avocado, ½ papaya lengthwise and place on either side of shrimp. (Note: The above salad can be topped with the dill sauce on page 114 or with the following curry topping.)

Curry Topping
⅓ cup safflower mayonnaise
2 heaping tsp. plain low-fat yogurt
2 tsp. curry powder
Squeeze lemon to taste.

This week covers _____ , _____ , _____ , to _____ , _____ , _____ .
month   day   year   month   day   year

Monday	E X E R C I S E	Activity _____ _____ Time _____ Distance _____ Pace _____ Effort: ☐ Easy ☐ Moderate ☐ Hard ☐ Extreme	Remarks (fitness): _____ _____ _____ Remarks (personal): _____ _____ _____
Resting Pulse Rate / **Weight At Rising**			

Tuesday	E X E R C I S E	Activity _____ _____ Time _____ Distance _____ Pace _____ Effort: ☐ Easy ☐ Moderate ☐ Hard ☐ Extreme	Remarks (fitness): _____ _____ _____ Remarks (personal): _____ _____ _____
Resting Pulse Rate / **Weight At Rising**			

Wednesday	E X E R C I S E	Activity _____ _____ Time _____ Distance _____ Pace _____ Effort: ☐ Easy ☐ Moderate ☐ Hard ☐ Extreme	Remarks (fitness): _____ _____ _____ Remarks (personal): _____ _____ _____
Resting Pulse Rate / **Weight At Rising**			

Thursday	E X E R C I S E	Activity _____ _____ Time _____ Distance _____ Pace _____ Effort: ☐ Easy ☐ Moderate ☐ Hard ☐ Extreme	Remarks (fitness): _____ _____ _____ Remarks (personal): _____ _____ _____
Resting Pulse Rate / **Weight At Rising**			

Friday	E X E R C I S E	Activity _____ _____ Time _____ Distance _____ Pace _____ Effort: ☐ Easy ☐ Moderate ☐ Hard ☐ Extreme	Remarks (fitness): _____ _____ _____ Remarks (personal): _____ _____ _____
Resting Pulse Rate / **Weight At Rising**			

Saturday	E X E R C I S E	Activity _____ _____ Time _____ Distance _____ Pace _____ Effort: ☐ Easy ☐ Moderate ☐ Hard ☐ Extreme	Remarks (fitness): _____ _____ _____ Remarks (personal): _____ _____ _____
Resting Pulse Rate / **Weight At Rising**			

Sunday	E X E R C I S E	Activity _____ _____ Time _____ Distance _____ Pace _____ Effort: ☐ Easy ☐ Moderate ☐ Hard ☐ Extreme	Remarks (fitness): _____ _____ _____ Remarks (personal): _____ _____ _____
Resting Pulse Rate / **Weight At Rising**			

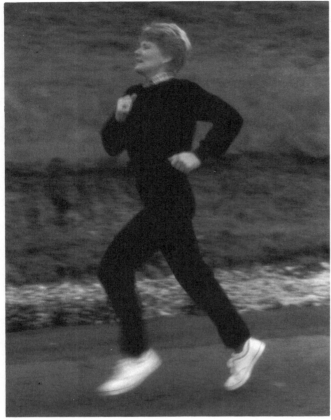

When you take up a fitness lifestyle, the only thing you stand to lose is what you didn't want anyway.

Goals for this week:

1. _____

2. _____

Goals for this month:

1. _____

2. _____

Running and Jogging

Recent national surveys indicate that there are about 30,000,000 people either running or jogging. That's a lot of people who've found one of the easiest forms of fitness available. If you are going to start running, remember these points: buy a good pair of running shoes, start easy enough so that you can hold a conversation while you run, and run only as long as it is comfortable.

Easy French Bread

2 pkgs. active dry yeast
½ cup warm water (110 degrees)
3 tbsp. honey
6 cups whole wheat pastry flour
¾ cup fortified whey powder or non-fat dry milk
1 tbsp. salt
2 cups warm water
2 tbsp. polyunsaturated oil

Dissolve yeast in warm water in 1 quart bowl, add honey; set aside to bubble. Combine all dry ingredients in large bowl; mix well. Add remaining water and oil to yeast mixture and pour into dry ingredients. Mix until smooth, adding ½ cup more flour to reach kneading consistency. Knead 3 minutes. Divide dough in half; form 2 loaves and place on greased cookie sheet. Cut 3 diagonal slashes across top and let rise. Bake at 450 degrees for 45 minutes. Remove from pans to cool.

Courtesy of The Whey Lovers' Cookbook

This week covers _____ , _____ , _____ , **to** _____ , _____ , _____ .

month   day   year   month   day   year

Monday	E X E R C I S E	Activity _____ _____ Time _____ Distance _____ Pace _____ Effort: ☐ Easy ☐ Moderate ☐ Hard ☐ Extreme	Remarks (fitness): _____ _____ _____ Remarks (personal): _____ _____ _____
Resting Pulse Rate / **Weight At Rising**			

Tuesday	E X E R C I S E	Activity _____ _____ Time _____ Distance _____ Pace _____ Effort: ☐ Easy ☐ Moderate ☐ Hard ☐ Extreme	Remarks (fitness): _____ _____ _____ Remarks (personal): _____ _____ _____
Resting Pulse Rate / **Weight At Rising**			

Wednesday	E X E R C I S E	Activity _____ _____ Time _____ Distance _____ Pace _____ Effort: ☐ Easy ☐ Moderate ☐ Hard ☐ Extreme	Remarks (fitness): _____ _____ _____ Remarks (personal): _____ _____ _____
Resting Pulse Rate / **Weight At Rising**			

Thursday	E X E R C I S E	Activity _____ _____ Time _____ Distance _____ Pace _____ Effort: ☐ Easy ☐ Moderate ☐ Hard ☐ Extreme	Remarks (fitness): _____ _____ _____ Remarks (personal): _____ _____ _____
Resting Pulse Rate / **Weight At Rising**			

Friday	E X E R C I S E	Activity _____ _____ Time _____ Distance _____ Pace _____ Effort: ☐ Easy ☐ Moderate ☐ Hard ☐ Extreme	Remarks (fitness): _____ _____ _____ Remarks (personal): _____ _____ _____
Resting Pulse Rate / **Weight At Rising**			

Saturday	E X E R C I S E	Activity _____ _____ Time _____ Distance _____ Pace _____ Effort: ☐ Easy ☐ Moderate ☐ Hard ☐ Extreme	Remarks (fitness): _____ _____ _____ Remarks (personal): _____ _____ _____
Resting Pulse Rate / **Weight At Rising**			

Sunday	E X E R C I S E	Activity _____ _____ Time _____ Distance _____ Pace _____ Effort: ☐ Easy ☐ Moderate ☐ Hard ☐ Extreme	Remarks (fitness): _____ _____ _____ Remarks (personal): _____ _____ _____
Resting Pulse Rate / **Weight At Rising**			

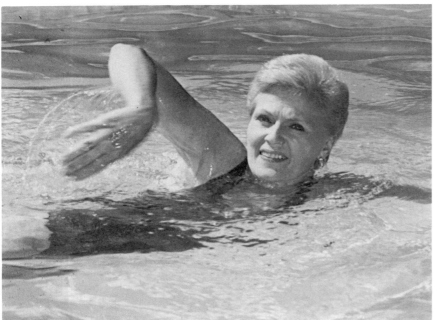

Swimming in Pool
Swimming is one of the most basic, and one of the best all-around exercises you can do. And, because you do it in the water, there is no harmful impacting, or traumatic beating that your body must take. It is an excellent aerobic sport and is something that can literally be learned by anyone. Highly recommended.

Goals for this week:

1. _____
2. _____

Goals for this month:

1. _____
2. _____

They say it takes 46 days from the time you begin a fitness program until you become reasonably fit. Considering the years of unfitness leading up to it, that seems like a pretty good deal.

Stuffed Mushrooms

2 bunches fresh spinach or
1 pkg. frozen chopped spinach
1 cup yogurt or mock sour cream
½ cup grated cheddar cheese
½ cup grated Jack cheese
½ cup grated Parmesan
¼ cup green chopped onions
½ tsp. Italian herb seasoning
garlic powder or freshly chopped
  garlic

Put the above over 2 cups fresh washed mushrooms in a 29-inch baking dish.
Second layer:
1 lb. ground beef or ground turkey
½ cup sliced green onions
1 tbsp. seasoning salt

Top with grated cheddar, Jack and Parmesan cheese and (optional) nutmeg. Bake in 350 degree oven for 25 minutes.

This week covers _____ , _____ , _____ , **to** _____ , _____ , _____ .
month   day   year   month   day   year

| **Monday** | E X E R C I S E | Activity _____
 _____
 Time _____
 Distance _____
 Pace _____
 Effort: ☐ Easy ☐ Moderate
 ☐ Hard ☐ Extreme | Remarks (fitness): _____
 _____
 _____
 Remarks (personal): _____
 _____
 _____ |
| Resting Pulse Rate | Weight At Rising | | |

| **Tuesday** | E X E R C I S E | Activity _____
 _____
 Time _____
 Distance _____
 Pace _____
 Effort: ☐ Easy ☐ Moderate
 ☐ Hard ☐ Extreme | Remarks (fitness): _____
 _____
 _____
 Remarks (personal): _____
 _____
 _____ |
| Resting Pulse Rate | Weight At Rising | | |

| **Wednesday** | E X E R C I S E | Activity _____
 _____
 Time _____
 Distance _____
 Pace _____
 Effort: ☐ Easy ☐ Moderate
 ☐ Hard ☐ Extreme | Remarks (fitness): _____
 _____
 _____
 Remarks (personal): _____
 _____
 _____ |
| Resting Pulse Rate | Weight At Rising | | |

| **Thursday** | E X E R C I S E | Activity _____
 _____
 Time _____
 Distance _____
 Pace _____
 Effort: ☐ Easy ☐ Moderate
 ☐ Hard ☐ Extreme | Remarks (fitness): _____
 _____
 _____
 Remarks (personal): _____
 _____
 _____ |
| Resting Pulse Rate | Weight At Rising | | |

| **Friday** | E X E R C I S E | Activity _____
 _____
 Time _____
 Distance _____
 Pace _____
 Effort: ☐ Easy ☐ Moderate
 ☐ Hard ☐ Extreme | Remarks (fitness): _____
 _____
 _____
 Remarks (personal): _____
 _____
 _____ |
| Resting Pulse Rate | Weight At Rising | | |

| **Saturday** | E X E R C I S E | Activity _____
 _____
 Time _____
 Distance _____
 Pace _____
 Effort: ☐ Easy ☐ Moderate
 ☐ Hard ☐ Extreme | Remarks (fitness): _____
 _____
 _____
 Remarks (personal): _____
 _____
 _____ |
| Resting Pulse Rate | Weight At Rising | | |

| **Sunday** | E X E R C I S E | Activity _____
 _____
 Time _____
 Distance _____
 Pace _____
 Effort: ☐ Easy ☐ Moderate
 ☐ Hard ☐ Extreme | Remarks (fitness): _____
 _____
 _____
 Remarks (personal): _____
 _____
 _____ |
| Resting Pulse Rate | Weight At Rising | | |

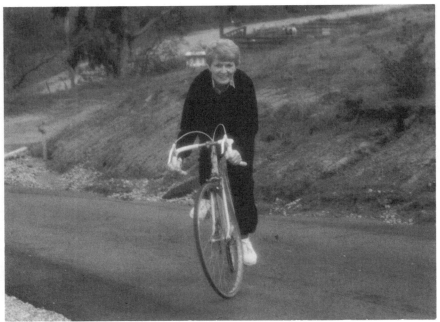

Riding a Bike
I can still vividly remember how much fun I had riding a bicycle as a child. Quite a bit of that fun comes back every time I get back on a bike. If you ride your bike with a regular cadence, you'll aerobically help yourself become more fit. In this picture, I'm trying to work my way up our driveway, which is pretty steep. Now that's a workout!

Goals for this week:
1. _____
2. _____

Goals for this month:
1. _____
2. _____

Even if being fit did not add an extra minute to your lifespan, it sure makes the available minutes a lot fuller.

Yellow Squash Casserole

2 lbs. crookneck yellow squash, thinly sliced
1 large onion, sliced in half moons
¼ lb. mushrooms, sliced
4 garlic cloves, minced
2 eggs, beaten
1 pt. lowfat cottage cheese
8 oz. Jack cheese, grated
4 tsp. oil
thyme
garlic powder
Parmesan cheese

Sauté garlic and onions in oil, about one minute. Add squash and lightly sauté. Remove from heat. In a casserole dish, spread a layer using half of the vegetables. Sprinkle with herbs and Parmesan. Then spread a layer using all of the cottage cheese. Next sprinkle on half of the grated cheese. Cover with remaining vegetables and eggs, then the rest of the cheese. Sprinkle with thyme and Parmesan. Bake in oven at 350 for 30 minutes.

This week covers _____ , _____ , _____ , **to** _____ , _____ , _____ .

month   day   year   month   day   year

Monday	E X E R C I S E	Activity _____ _____ Time _____ Distance _____ Pace _____ Effort: ☐ Easy ☐ Moderate ☐ Hard ☐ Extreme	Remarks (fitness): _____ _____ _____ Remarks (personal): _____ _____

Resting Pulse Rate	**Weight At Rising**

Tuesday	E X E R C I S E	Activity _____ _____ Time _____ Distance _____ Pace _____ Effort: ☐ Easy ☐ Moderate ☐ Hard ☐ Extreme	Remarks (fitness): _____ _____ Remarks (personal): _____ _____

Resting Pulse Rate	**Weight At Rising**

Wednesday	E X E R C I S E	Activity _____ _____ Time _____ Distance _____ Pace _____ Effort: ☐ Easy ☐ Moderate ☐ Hard ☐ Extreme	Remarks (fitness): _____ _____ Remarks (personal): _____ _____

Resting Pulse Rate	**Weight At Rising**

Thursday	E X E R C I S E	Activity _____ _____ Time _____ Distance _____ Pace _____ Effort: ☐ Easy ☐ Moderate ☐ Hard ☐ Extreme	Remarks (fitness): _____ _____ Remarks (personal): _____ _____

Resting Pulse Rate	**Weight At Rising**

Friday	E X E R C I S E	Activity _____ _____ Time _____ Distance _____ Pace _____ Effort: ☐ Easy ☐ Moderate ☐ Hard ☐ Extreme	Remarks (fitness): _____ _____ Remarks (personal): _____ _____

Resting Pulse Rate	**Weight At Rising**

Saturday	E X E R C I S E	Activity _____ _____ Time _____ Distance _____ Pace _____ Effort: ☐ Easy ☐ Moderate ☐ Hard ☐ Extreme	Remarks (fitness): _____ _____ Remarks (personal): _____ _____

Resting Pulse Rate	**Weight At Rising**

Sunday	E X E R C I S E	Activity _____ _____ Time _____ Distance _____ Pace _____ Effort: ☐ Easy ☐ Moderate ☐ Hard ☐ Extreme	Remarks (fitness): _____ _____ Remarks (personal): _____ _____

Resting Pulse Rate	**Weight At Rising**

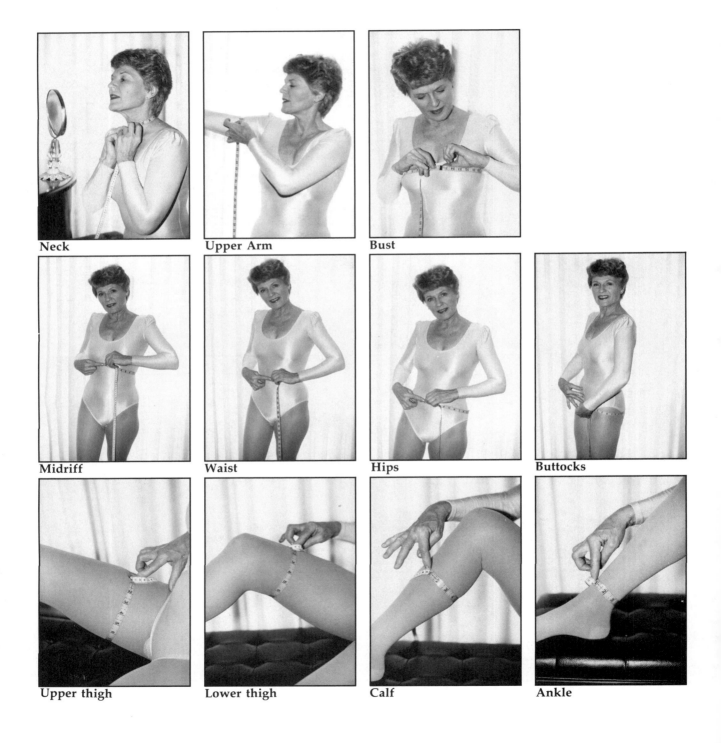

Neck

Upper Arm

Bust

Midriff

Waist

Hips

Buttocks

Upper thigh

Lower thigh

Calf

Ankle

Neck

Upper Arm

Bust

Midriff

Waist

Hips

Buttocks

Upper thigh

Lower thigh

Calf

Ankle

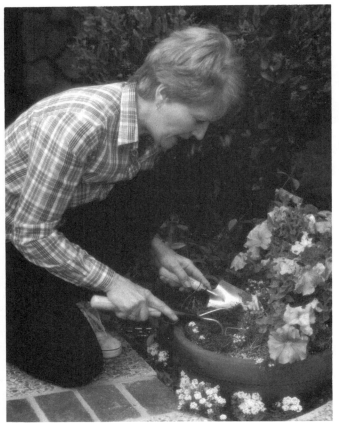

If, as they say, there's a lid for every pot, there's an aerobic sport for each of us. The problem is, once you've tried them all, it's difficult deciding which one you like most.

Goals for this week:
1. _____
2. _____
Goals for this month:
1. _____
2. _____

Gardening
Don't overlook the fact that many activities around the house, whether they are work or hobbies, can offer opportunities to bend, stretch and exercise. Don't overlook hobbies and activities that require a little work as relaxation outlets. Many of us have jobs that offer precious little physical activity, so if you can get an opportunity to work in the garden or pursue some other hobby outside, take the opportunity to do so.

Seaweed Soup
2½ cups chicken broth (homemade stock preferred)
1 pkg. seaweed, torn in pieces
½ cup chicken pieces (chopped)
1 chopped green onion
½ cup fresh or canned mushrooms (chopped)
½ cup water chestnuts (chopped)
1 egg, beaten

Heat broth in saucepan, adding ingredients. Lastly add seaweed, which has been presoaked in water and dried, and egg. Quickly mix and serve.

This week covers _____ , _____ , _____ , **to** _____ , _____ , _____ .
month   day   year   month   day   year

Monday

Resting Pulse Rate	Weight At Rising

EXERCISE

Activity _____
_____
Time _____
Distance _____
Pace _____
Effort: ☐ Easy ☐ Moderate
☐ Hard ☐ Extreme

Remarks (fitness): _____
_____
Remarks (personal): _____
_____
_____

Tuesday

Resting Pulse Rate	Weight At Rising

EXERCISE

Activity _____
_____
Time _____
Distance _____
Pace _____
Effort: ☐ Easy ☐ Moderate
☐ Hard ☐ Extreme

Remarks (fitness): _____
_____
Remarks (personal): _____
_____
_____

Wednesday

Resting Pulse Rate	Weight At Rising

EXERCISE

Activity _____
_____
Time _____
Distance _____
Pace _____
Effort: ☐ Easy ☐ Moderate
☐ Hard ☐ Extreme

Remarks (fitness): _____
_____
Remarks (personal): _____
_____
_____

Thursday

Resting Pulse Rate	Weight At Rising

EXERCISE

Activity _____
_____
Time _____
Distance _____
Pace _____
Effort: ☐ Easy ☐ Moderate
☐ Hard ☐ Extreme

Remarks (fitness): _____
_____
Remarks (personal): _____
_____

Friday

Resting Pulse Rate	Weight At Rising

EXERCISE

Activity _____
_____
Time _____
Distance _____
Pace _____
Effort: ☐ Easy ☐ Moderate
☐ Hard ☐ Extreme

Remarks (fitness): _____
_____
Remarks (personal): _____
_____

Saturday

Resting Pulse Rate	Weight At Rising

EXERCISE

Activity _____
_____
Time _____
Distance _____
Pace _____
Effort: ☐ Easy ☐ Moderate
☐ Hard ☐ Extreme

Remarks (fitness): _____
_____
Remarks (personal): _____
_____

Sunday

Resting Pulse Rate	Weight At Rising

EXERCISE

Activity _____
_____
Time _____
Distance _____
Pace _____
Effort: ☐ Easy ☐ Moderate
☐ Hard ☐ Extreme

Remarks (fitness): _____
_____
Remarks (personal): _____
_____

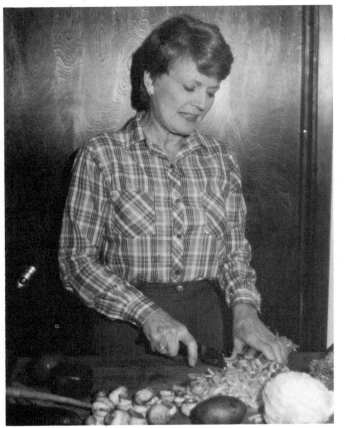

An investment in fitness today offers dividends and bene-*fit* for the rest of your life.

Goals for this week:
1. _____
2. _____
Goals for this month:
1. _____
2. _____

Food

One of the most important elements in a fitness program is good nutrition. You should not have to diet, which is an unnatural act, if you are active. You should watch what you eat, certainly, and make sure to eat as much nutritious food as possible, but that doesn't mean that you must adopt some complicated or mystical nutrition routine. Jack and I avoid white flour and white sugar, eat mainly chicken, fish and turkey, and do not eat in between meals. Moderation is our motto. I also avoid the word diet; I suggest you go on a ''way of life'' rather than a diet. To me diet means temporary.

Scrambled Eggs and Salsa

1 zucchini, chopped
2-3 mushrooms, chopped (optional)
1 green onion, tops chopped
1 tomato, chopped
1 heart of celery stalk, chopped
4 eggs

Sauté the vegetables in 1 tbsp. oil; add tomato last. Scramble 4 eggs in separate frying pan. Serve eggs in individual platters, garnish with parsley and top with above salsa.

This week covers _____ , _____ , _____ , to _____ , _____ , _____ .
               month   day   year   month   day   year

Monday

Resting Pulse Rate	Weight At Rising

EXERCISE

Activity _____
_____
Time _____
Distance _____
Pace _____
Effort: ☐ Easy ☐ Moderate
        ☐ Hard ☐ Extreme

Remarks (fitness): _____
_____
_____
Remarks (personal): _____
_____
_____

Tuesday

Resting Pulse Rate	Weight At Rising

EXERCISE

Activity _____
_____
Time _____
Distance _____
Pace _____
Effort: ☐ Easy ☐ Moderate
        ☐ Hard ☐ Extreme

Remarks (fitness): _____
_____
_____
Remarks (personal): _____
_____
_____

Wednesday

Resting Pulse Rate	Weight At Rising

EXERCISE

Activity _____
_____
Time _____
Distance _____
Pace _____
Effort: ☐ Easy ☐ Moderate
        ☐ Hard ☐ Extreme

Remarks (fitness): _____
_____
_____
Remarks (personal): _____
_____
_____

Thursday

Resting Pulse Rate	Weight At Rising

EXERCISE

Activity _____
_____
Time _____
Distance _____
Pace _____
Effort: ☐ Easy ☐ Moderate
        ☐ Hard ☐ Extreme

Remarks (fitness): _____
_____
_____
Remarks (personal): _____
_____
_____

Friday

Resting Pulse Rate	Weight At Rising

EXERCISE

Activity _____
_____
Time _____
Distance _____
Pace _____
Effort: ☐ Easy ☐ Moderate
        ☐ Hard ☐ Extreme

Remarks (fitness): _____
_____
_____
Remarks (personal): _____
_____
_____

Saturday

Resting Pulse Rate	Weight At Rising

EXERCISE

Activity _____
_____
Time _____
Distance _____
Pace _____
Effort: ☐ Easy ☐ Moderate
        ☐ Hard ☐ Extreme

Remarks (fitness): _____
_____
_____
Remarks (personal): _____
_____
_____

Sunday

Resting Pulse Rate	Weight At Rising

EXERCISE

Activity _____
_____
Time _____
Distance _____
Pace _____
Effort: ☐ Easy ☐ Moderate
        ☐ Hard ☐ Extreme

Remarks (fitness): _____
_____
_____
Remarks (personal): _____
_____
_____

If you put off until tomorrow what you can do today, it is surprising how quickly tomorrow is upon you, and you're almost always too late to do anything about it.

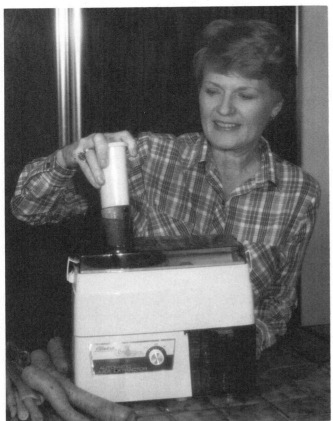

Juice Extractor
With some of the new gadgets available for the kitchen, cooking can be a real adventure. What I'm using here is a juice extractor. Jack and I really enjoy a good, nutritious glass of juice made from mixed vegetables.

Goals for this week:
1. _____
2. _____

Goals for this month:
1. _____
2. _____

Granola Bars

¼ cup raw honey
½ cup raw unsalted peanut butter
2 tbsp. margarine or safflower oil
1 tsp. vanilla
2 cups granola

Preheat oven to 350 degrees. Mix all the above ingredients together and spread in Pyrex pan, approximately ½-inch thickness. You may vary these bars by adding raisins, nuts, dates, sunflower seeds and/or coconut. Bake approximately 10 minutes. Allow to cool and cut into squares.

This week covers _____ , _____ , _____ , **to** _____ , _____ , _____ .
month   day   year   month   day   year

Monday

Resting Pulse Rate	Weight At Rising

E X E R C I S E

Activity _____

_____

Time _____

Distance _____

Pace _____

Effort: ☐ Easy ☐ Moderate ☐ Hard ☐ Extreme

Remarks (fitness): _____

_____

Remarks (personal): _____

_____

Tuesday

Resting Pulse Rate	Weight At Rising

E X E R C I S E

Activity _____

_____

Time _____

Distance _____

Pace _____

Effort: ☐ Easy ☐ Moderate ☐ Hard ☐ Extreme

Remarks (fitness): _____

_____

Remarks (personal): _____

_____

Wednesday

Resting Pulse Rate	Weight At Rising

E X E R C I S E

Activity _____

_____

Time _____

Distance _____

Pace _____

Effort: ☐ Easy ☐ Moderate ☐ Hard ☐ Extreme

Remarks (fitness): _____

_____

Remarks (personal): _____

_____

Thursday

Resting Pulse Rate	Weight At Rising

E X E R C I S E

Activity _____

_____

Time _____

Distance _____

Pace _____

Effort: ☐ Easy ☐ Moderate ☐ Hard ☐ Extreme

Remarks (fitness): _____

_____

Remarks (personal): _____

_____

Friday

Resting Pulse Rate	Weight At Rising

E X E R C I S E

Activity _____

_____

Time _____

Distance _____

Pace _____

Effort: ☐ Easy ☐ Moderate ☐ Hard ☐ Extreme

Remarks (fitness): _____

_____

Remarks (personal): _____

_____

Saturday

Resting Pulse Rate	Weight At Rising

E X E R C I S E

Activity _____

Time _____

Distance _____

Pace _____

Effort: ☐ Easy ☐ Moderate ☐ Hard ☐ Extreme

Remarks (fitness): _____

_____

Remarks (personal): _____

_____

Sunday

Resting Pulse Rate	Weight At Rising

E X E R C I S E

Activity _____

_____

Time _____

Distance _____

Pace _____

Effort: ☐ Easy ☐ Moderate ☐ Hard ☐ Extreme

Remarks (fitness): _____

_____

Remarks (personal): _____

_____

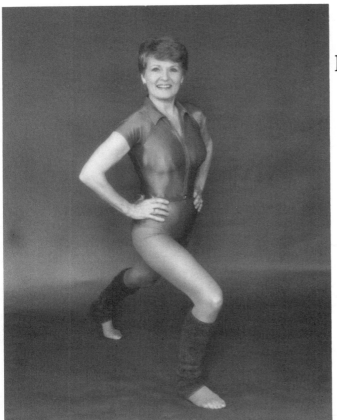

A good rule to remember when contemplating the limits your fitness will reach is that there are no limits.

Goals for this week:

1. _____

2. _____

Goals for this month:

1. _____

2. _____

Forward Leg Lunges

I feel that Leg Lunges help keep my hips and thighs tight and firm. If done properly, they can also do the same for you. I really enjoy doing them first thing in the morning along with my swings; however, being advanced, I jump into them, which makes a great cardio-vascular exercise. Stand erect, hands on hips or chair for balance. Lunge forward similar to a fencing pose. Step back and lunge forward on the opposite leg.

Leftover Potato Scramble

1 boiled potato with skin, chopped coarse

1 small bell pepper, chopped fine

2-3 eggs, beaten

1 tbsp. chopped onion (optional)

Preheat skillet with 1 tbsp. oil or more, as needed, and sauté peppers. Then add potatoes and sauté slightly, lastly adding eggs. Stir until desired consistency. Turn into plate.

This week covers _____ , _____ , _____ , to _____ , _____ , _____ .
month　　　　day　　　　year　　　　　month　　　　day　　　　year

Monday	E	Activity _____	Remarks (fitness): _____
Resting Pulse Rate / **Weight At Rising**	X E R C I S E	_____ Time _____ Distance _____ Pace _____ Effort: ☐ Easy ☐ Moderate 　　　　 ☐ Hard ☐ Extreme	_____ _____ Remarks (personal): _____ _____ _____

Tuesday	E	Activity _____	Remarks (fitness): _____
Resting Pulse Rate / **Weight At Rising**	X E R C I S E	_____ Time _____ Distance _____ Pace _____ Effort: ☐ Easy ☐ Moderate 　　　　 ☐ Hard ☐ Extreme	_____ _____ Remarks (personal): _____ _____ _____

Wednesday	E	Activity _____	Remarks (fitness): _____
Resting Pulse Rate / **Weight At Rising**	X E R C I S E	_____ Time _____ Distance _____ Pace _____ Effort: ☐ Easy ☐ Moderate 　　　　 ☐ Hard ☐ Extreme	_____ _____ Remarks (personal): _____ _____ _____

Thursday	E	Activity _____	Remarks (fitness): _____
Resting Pulse Rate / **Weight At Rising**	X E R C I S E	_____ Time _____ Distance _____ Pace _____ Effort: ☐ Easy ☐ Moderate 　　　　 ☐ Hard ☐ Extreme	_____ _____ Remarks (personal): _____ _____ _____

Friday	E	Activity _____	Remarks (fitness): _____
Resting Pulse Rate / **Weight At Rising**	X E R C I S E	_____ Time _____ Distance _____ Pace _____ Effort: ☐ Easy ☐ Moderate 　　　　 ☐ Hard ☐ Extreme	_____ _____ Remarks (personal): _____ _____ _____

Saturday	E	Activity _____	Remarks (fitness): _____
Resting Pulse Rate / **Weight At Rising**	X E R C I S E	_____ Time _____ Distance _____ Pace _____ Effort: ☐ Easy ☐ Moderate 　　　　 ☐ Hard ☐ Extreme	_____ _____ Remarks (personal): _____ _____ _____

Sunday	E	Activity _____	Remarks (fitness): _____
Resting Pulse Rate / **Weight At Rising**	X E R C I S E	_____ Time _____ Distance _____ Pace _____ Effort: ☐ Easy ☐ Moderate 　　　　 ☐ Hard ☐ Extreme	_____ _____ Remarks (personal): _____ _____ _____

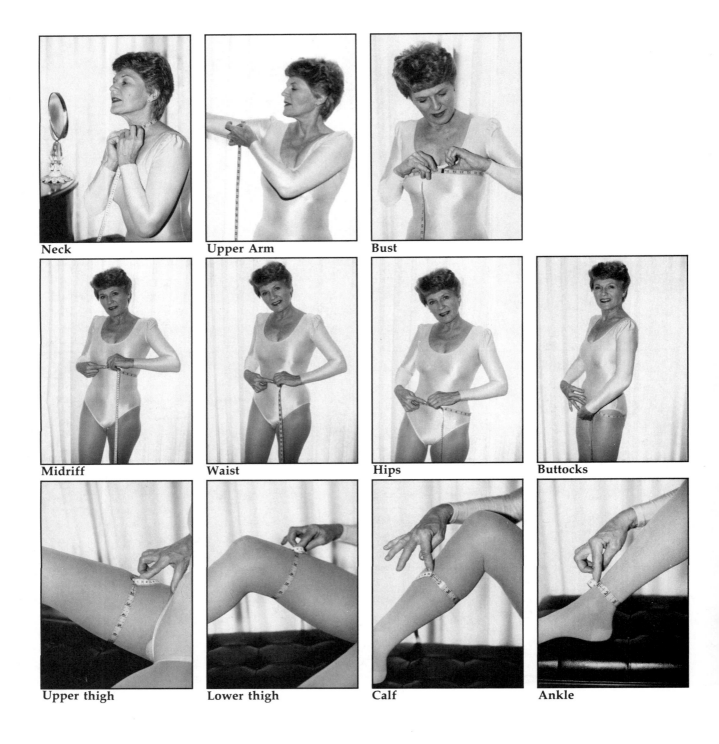

Neck

Upper Arm

Bust

Midriff

Waist

Hips

Buttocks

Upper thigh

Lower thigh

Calf

Ankle

Neck

Upper Arm

Bust

Midriff

Waist

Hips

Buttocks

Upper thigh

Lower thigh

Calf

Ankle

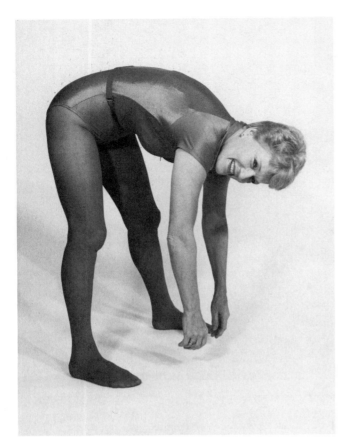

Don't wait for free time to come along to allow you to get your fitness program going. Fit people are active people, and they don't have time to get fit—they *make* time for fitness.

Goals for this week:

1. _____

2. _____

Goals for this month:

1. _____

2. _____

Rag Doll Relaxer

Another exercise that is terrific first thing in the morning is the good ol' Rag Doll Stretch. With feet shoulder-width apart, bend at the waist, legs straight, try to keep your back flat and allow your arms to hang loosely toward the floor. Allow gravity to do the work. Don't bounce. Just hang. Feel your body stretching? Aaaaaaaah!

Oatmeal Cookies

¾ **cup safflower oil**

1½ **cups honey**

1 **egg**

¼ **cup orange juice**

1 **tsp. vanilla**

3 **cups oats, uncooked**

1 **cup whole wheat flour (you may combine wheat germ)**

1 **tsp. salt**

½ **tsp. soda**

Preheat oven to 350 degrees. Beat together oil, honey, egg, juice and vanilla until creamy. Add combined remaining ingredients; mix well. Drop by rounded teaspoonfuls onto greased cookie sheet. Bake at 350 degrees for 12-15 minutes. (For variety, add chopped nuts, raisins, chocolate or carob chips or coconut.)

This week covers _____ , _____ , _____ , **to** _____ , _____ , _____ .
month   day   year   month   day   year

Monday

Resting Pulse Rate	Weight At Rising

EXERCISE

Activity _____
_____
Time _____
Distance _____
Pace _____
Effort: ☐ Easy   ☐ Moderate
       ☐ Hard   ☐ Extreme

Remarks (fitness): _____
_____
Remarks (personal): _____
_____
_____

Tuesday

Resting Pulse Rate	Weight At Rising

EXERCISE

Activity _____
_____
Time _____
Distance _____
Pace _____
Effort: ☐ Easy   ☐ Moderate
       ☐ Hard   ☐ Extreme

Remarks (fitness): _____
_____
Remarks (personal): _____
_____
_____

Wednesday

Resting Pulse Rate	Weight At Rising

EXERCISE

Activity _____
_____
Time _____
Distance _____
Pace _____
Effort: ☐ Easy   ☐ Moderate
       ☐ Hard   ☐ Extreme

Remarks (fitness): _____
_____
Remarks (personal): _____
_____
_____

Thursday

Resting Pulse Rate	Weight At Rising

EXERCISE

Activity _____
_____
Time _____
Distance _____
Pace _____
Effort: ☐ Easy   ☐ Moderate
       ☐ Hard   ☐ Extreme

Remarks (fitness): _____
_____
Remarks (personal): _____
_____
_____

Friday

Resting Pulse Rate	Weight At Rising

EXERCISE

Activity _____
_____
Time _____
Distance _____
Pace _____
Effort: ☐ Easy   ☐ Moderate
       ☐ Hard   ☐ Extreme

Remarks (fitness): _____
_____
Remarks (personal): _____
_____
_____

Saturday

Resting Pulse Rate	Weight At Rising

EXERCISE

Activity _____
_____
Time _____
Distance _____
Pace _____
Effort: ☐ Easy   ☐ Moderate
       ☐ Hard   ☐ Extreme

Remarks (fitness): _____
_____
Remarks (personal): _____
_____
_____

Sunday

Resting Pulse Rate	Weight At Rising

EXERCISE

Activity _____
_____
Time _____
Distance _____
Pace _____
Effort: ☐ Easy   ☐ Moderate
       ☐ Hard   ☐ Extreme

Remarks (fitness): _____
_____
Remarks (personal): _____
_____
_____

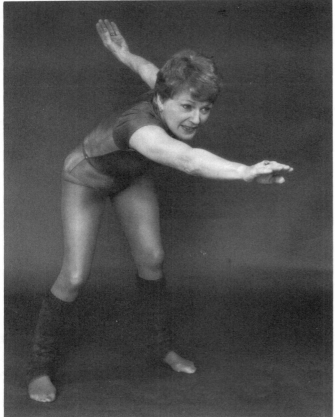

Recent studies have indicated that the aerobically fit person metabolizes more calories even during sleep than the unfit person does; fitness is full-time.

Goals for this week:
1. _____
2. _____

Goals for this month:
1. _____
2. _____

The Swimmer
This exercise helps the shoulders, back of arms, bra hangover, waistline and round shoulders. Bend over at the waist, feet shoulder-width apart, bend knees, bring arm up toward your ear as in a swimming motion. Pretend you are swimming. Try to keep horizontal to the floor with your head up while doing this exercise. Wonderful for your posture, too.

Tofu Rice Pudding

12 oz. mashed tofu
1 to 1½ cups cooked brown rice
¾ cup nonfat dry milk or
   whey powder
3 tbsp. honey
½ tsp. cinnamon
⅛ tsp. cloves
¼ cup raisins
1 tsp. safflower oil
3 tbsp. granola

Combine tofu, rice, milk, honey, spices and raisins in a large bowl. Mix well. Coat a quart size baking dish or bowl with oil. Spoon in tofu mixture. Sprinkle with granola. Bake 45 minutes or until set in 350 degree oven.

This week covers _____ , _____ , _____ , to _____ , _____ , _____ .
month   day   year   month   day   year

Monday

Resting Pulse Rate	Weight At Rising

EXERCISE

Activity _____
_____
Time _____
Distance _____
Pace _____
Effort: ☐ Easy ☐ Moderate ☐ Hard ☐ Extreme

Remarks (fitness): _____
_____
_____
Remarks (personal): _____
_____
_____

Tuesday

Resting Pulse Rate	Weight At Rising

EXERCISE

Activity _____
_____
Time _____
Distance _____
Pace _____
Effort: ☐ Easy ☐ Moderate ☐ Hard ☐ Extreme

Remarks (fitness): _____
_____
_____
Remarks (personal): _____
_____
_____

Wednesday

Resting Pulse Rate	Weight At Rising

EXERCISE

Activity _____
_____
Time _____
Distance _____
Pace _____
Effort: ☐ Easy ☐ Moderate ☐ Hard ☐ Extreme

Remarks (fitness): _____
_____
_____
Remarks (personal): _____
_____
_____

Thursday

Resting Pulse Rate	Weight At Rising

EXERCISE

Activity _____
_____
Time _____
Distance _____
Pace _____
Effort: ☐ Easy ☐ Moderate ☐ Hard ☐ Extreme

Remarks (fitness): _____
_____
_____
Remarks (personal): _____
_____
_____

Friday

Resting Pulse Rate	Weight At Rising

EXERCISE

Activity _____
_____
Time _____
Distance _____
Pace _____
Effort: ☐ Easy ☐ Moderate ☐ Hard ☐ Extreme

Remarks (fitness): _____
_____
_____
Remarks (personal): _____
_____
_____

Saturday

Resting Pulse Rate	Weight At Rising

EXERCISE

Activity _____
_____
Time _____
Distance _____
Pace _____
Effort: ☐ Easy ☐ Moderate ☐ Hard ☐ Extreme

Remarks (fitness): _____
_____
_____
Remarks (personal): _____
_____
_____

Sunday

Resting Pulse Rate	Weight At Rising

EXERCISE

Activity _____
_____
Time _____
Distance _____
Pace _____
Effort: ☐ Easy ☐ Moderate ☐ Hard ☐ Extreme

Remarks (fitness): _____
_____
_____
Remarks (personal): _____
_____
_____

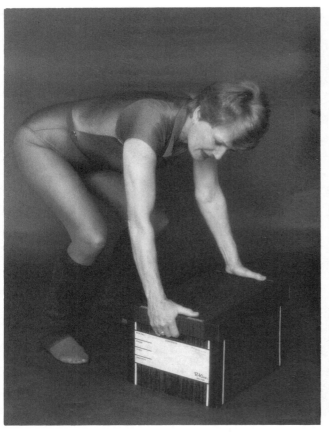

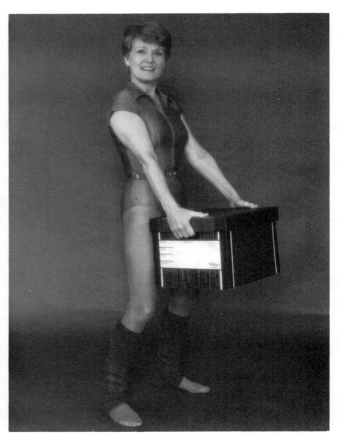

How to Lift a Heavy Object
The most important thing to remember, when you are lifting a heavy object, is to bend your knees, keeping your back flat. Keep the weight close into your thighs as much as possible so that your thigh muscles will do the lifting and take the strain off your back.

Goals for this week:
1. _____
2. _____

Goals for this month:
1. _____
2. _____

Carrot Raisin Pineapple Salad

2 cups grated carrots
½ cup raisins or currants
½ cup pineapple chunks
¼ cup honey
¼ cup oil
¼ lemon juice
¼ cup chopped walnuts

Toss all together, place on lettuce leaves. Grated apple can also be added.

Being fit does not cure any diseases. It merely works to prevent them.

This week covers _____ , _____ , _____ , **to** _____ , _____ , _____ .
month   day   year   month   day   year

Monday	E X E R C I S E	Activity _____ _____ Time _____ Distance _____ Pace _____ Effort: ☐ Easy ☐ Moderate ☐ Hard ☐ Extreme	Remarks (fitness): _____ _____ _____ Remarks (personal): _____ _____ _____
Resting Pulse Rate / **Weight At Rising**			
Tuesday	E X E R C I S E	Activity _____ _____ Time _____ Distance _____ Pace _____ Effort: ☐ Easy ☐ Moderate ☐ Hard ☐ Extreme	Remarks (fitness): _____ _____ _____ Remarks (personal): _____ _____ _____
Resting Pulse Rate / **Weight At Rising**			
Wednesday	E X E R C I S E	Activity _____ _____ Time _____ Distance _____ Pace _____ Effort: ☐ Easy ☐ Moderate ☐ Hard ☐ Extreme	Remarks (fitness): _____ _____ _____ Remarks (personal): _____ _____ _____
Resting Pulse Rate / **Weight At Rising**			
Thursday	E X E R C I S E	Activity _____ _____ Time _____ Distance _____ Pace _____ Effort: ☐ Easy ☐ Moderate ☐ Hard ☐ Extreme	Remarks (fitness): _____ _____ _____ Remarks (personal): _____ _____ _____
Resting Pulse Rate / **Weight At Rising**			
Friday	E X E R C I S E	Activity _____ _____ Time _____ Distance _____ Pace _____ Effort: ☐ Easy ☐ Moderate ☐ Hard ☐ Extreme	Remarks (fitness): _____ _____ _____ Remarks (personal): _____ _____ _____
Resting Pulse Rate / **Weight At Rising**			
Saturday	E X E R C I S E	Activity _____ _____ Time _____ Distance _____ Pace _____ Effort: ☐ Easy ☐ Moderate ☐ Hard ☐ Extreme	Remarks (fitness): _____ _____ _____ Remarks (personal): _____ _____ _____
Resting Pulse Rate / **Weight At Rising**			
Sunday	E X E R C I S E	Activity _____ _____ Time _____ Distance _____ Pace _____ Effort: ☐ Easy ☐ Moderate ☐ Hard ☐ Extreme	Remarks (fitness): _____ _____ _____ Remarks (personal): _____ _____ _____
Resting Pulse Rate / **Weight At Rising**			

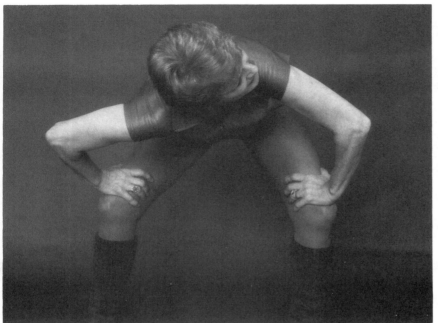

Neck Rotator
This is a very good exercise for your neck and shoulders, and I like to use it after I've had a hard day at the office, or when I get a little stiff in the upper body. If you tend to get tense and it settles in your neck and shoulders, this one is for you. Stand in a wide stance, bend forward at the waist with your hands on your knees, try to look up at the ceiling. Turn your head slowly from side to side. It feels wonderful.

Goals for this week:
1. _____
2. _____

Goals for this month:
1. _____
2. _____

The biggest barrier to fitness, whether you're just starting or whether you're contemplating today's workout, is inertia. Overcome that, and it's easy.

Squash Medley

Chop the following ingredients into bite-size pieces and sauté in safflower oil keeping them crisp.
1 large zucchini (or 2 small)
1 large summer squash (or 2 small)
1 large gooseneck yellow squash (or 2 small)
1 small onion or 2 green onions

Variation: Add ½ pound ground beef or ground turkey, seasoning to taste (salt, pepper, garlic and onion powder), sautéing until meat is cooked.

This week covers _____ , _____ , _____ , to _____ , _____ , _____ .
month   day   year   month   day   year

Monday

Resting Pulse Rate	Weight At Rising

E X E R C I S E

Activity _____
_____
Time _____
Distance _____
Pace _____
Effort: ☐ Easy ☐ Moderate
☐ Hard ☐ Extreme

Remarks (fitness): _____
_____
Remarks (personal): _____
_____

Tuesday

Resting Pulse Rate	Weight At Rising

E X E R C I S E

Activity _____
_____
Time _____
Distance _____
Pace _____
Effort: ☐ Easy ☐ Moderate
☐ Hard ☐ Extreme

Remarks (fitness): _____
_____
Remarks (personal): _____
_____

Wednesday

Resting Pulse Rate	Weight At Rising

E X E R C I S E

Activity _____
_____
Time _____
Distance _____
Pace _____
Effort: ☐ Easy ☐ Moderate
☐ Hard ☐ Extreme

Remarks (fitness): _____
_____
Remarks (personal): _____
_____

Thursday

Resting Pulse Rate	Weight At Rising

E X E R C I S E

Activity _____
_____
Time _____
Distance _____
Pace _____
Effort: ☐ Easy ☐ Moderate
☐ Hard ☐ Extreme

Remarks (fitness): _____
_____
Remarks (personal): _____
_____

Friday

Resting Pulse Rate	Weight At Rising

E X E R C I S E

Activity _____
_____
Time _____
Distance _____
Pace _____
Effort: ☐ Easy ☐ Moderate
☐ Hard ☐ Extreme

Remarks (fitness): _____
_____
Remarks (personal): _____
_____

Saturday

Resting Pulse Rate	Weight At Rising

E X E R C I S E

Activity _____
_____
Time _____
Distance _____
Pace _____
Effort: ☐ Easy ☐ Moderate
☐ Hard ☐ Extreme

Remarks (fitness): _____
_____
Remarks (personal): _____
_____

Sunday

Resting Pulse Rate	Weight At Rising

E X E R C I S E

Activity _____
Time _____
Distance _____
Pace _____
Effort: ☐ Easy ☐ Moderate
☐ Hard ☐ Extreme

Remarks (fitness): _____
_____
Remarks (personal): _____
_____

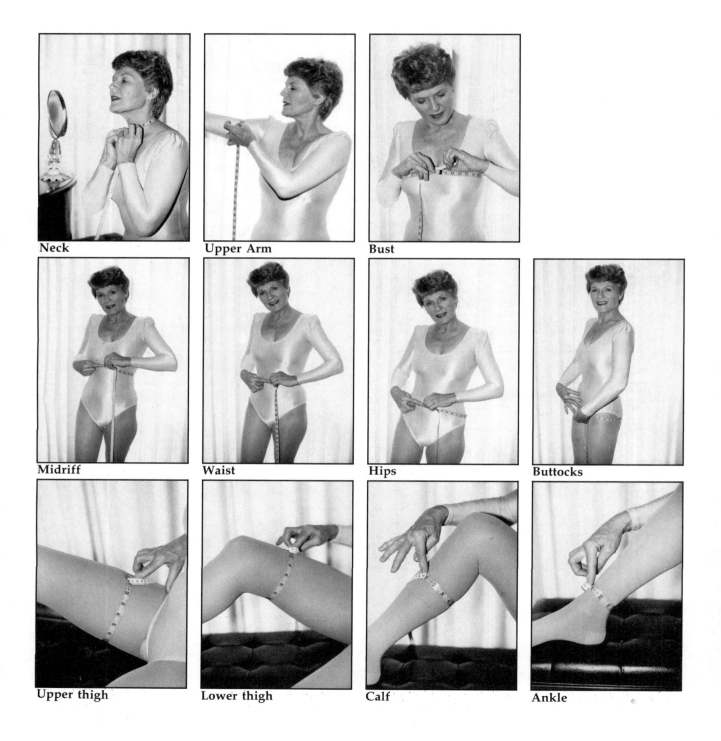

Neck

Upper Arm

Bust

Midriff

Waist

Hips

Buttocks

Upper thigh

Lower thigh

Calf

Ankle

Neck

Upper Arm

Bust

Midriff

Waist

Hips

Buttocks

Upper thigh

Lower thigh

Calf

Ankle

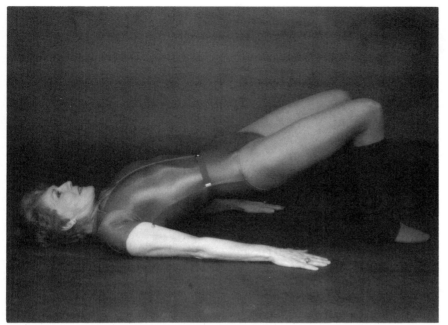

Arch Ups
This is a wonderful way to help firm, tighten and strengthen the back of the legs, back of the hips and lower back. Place your arms by your sides for support. Lie flat on your back, bend knees, feet flat on floor and raise hips up as high as possible.

Goals for this week:
1. _____
2. _____

Goals for this month:
1. _____
2. _____

Consider this: If you exercise one hour at a time, five days a week, you get 168 hours of benefit per week for an investment of five hours. What a bargain!

Beans with Peppers and Carrots

2 cups lima beans
4 cups water
1 tsp. sea salt
½ tsp. pepper
½ tsp. garlic powder
2 tbsp. safflower oil
1 onion, chopped
½ green pepper, chopped
½ red pepper, chopped
2 carrots, grated

Add beans, seasonings, oil, and onions to boiling water. Cover and simmer for 1½ hours, add more water if necessary. Add peppers and carrots and simmer until tender.

This week covers _____ , _____ , _____ , **to** _____ , _____ , _____ .
month   day   year   month   day   year

Monday

Resting Pulse Rate	Weight At Rising

EXERCISE

Activity _____
_____
Time _____
Distance _____
Pace _____
Effort: ☐ Easy ☐ Moderate ☐ Hard ☐ Extreme

Remarks (fitness): _____
_____
Remarks (personal): _____
_____

Tuesday

Resting Pulse Rate	Weight At Rising

EXERCISE

Activity _____
_____
Time _____
Distance _____
Pace _____
Effort: ☐ Easy ☐ Moderate ☐ Hard ☐ Extreme

Remarks (fitness): _____
_____
Remarks (personal): _____
_____

Wednesday

Resting Pulse Rate	Weight At Rising

EXERCISE

Activity _____
_____
Time _____
Distance _____
Pace _____
Effort: ☐ Easy ☐ Moderate ☐ Hard ☐ Extreme

Remarks (fitness): _____
_____
Remarks (personal): _____
_____

Thursday

Resting Pulse Rate	Weight At Rising

EXERCISE

Activity _____
_____
Time _____
Distance _____
Pace _____
Effort: ☐ Easy ☐ Moderate ☐ Hard ☐ Extreme

Remarks (fitness): _____
_____
Remarks (personal): _____
_____

Friday

Resting Pulse Rate	Weight At Rising

EXERCISE

Activity _____
_____
Time _____
Distance _____
Pace _____
Effort: ☐ Easy ☐ Moderate ☐ Hard ☐ Extreme

Remarks (fitness): _____
_____
Remarks (personal): _____
_____

Saturday

Resting Pulse Rate	Weight At Rising

EXERCISE

Activity _____
_____
Time _____
Distance _____
Pace _____
Effort: ☐ Easy ☐ Moderate ☐ Hard ☐ Extreme

Remarks (fitness): _____
_____
Remarks (personal): _____
_____

Sunday

Resting Pulse Rate	Weight At Rising

EXERCISE

Activity _____
_____
Time _____
Distance _____
Pace _____
Effort: ☐ Easy ☐ Moderate ☐ Hard ☐ Extreme

Remarks (fitness): _____
_____
Remarks (personal): _____
_____

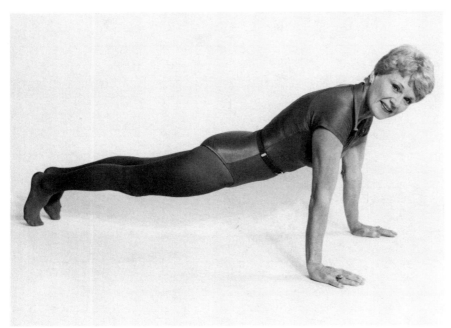

Standard Push-Up

The Standard Push-Up is more difficult than the push-up we discussed on page 36. Rise up on your toes and up on your arms, keeping your body perfectly straight. Let your arms do all the work. Lower yourself to the floor, touching the floor briefly with your chest. Push yourself back up. Repeat as many times as possible. Don't give up.

Goals for this week:

1. _____

2. _____

Goals for this month:

1. _____

2. _____

If you don't like to do anything halfway in life, don't get halfway through your life before you decide to get fit.

Brown Rice Cereal

4 oz. cooked brown rice
honey
raisins
½ to ¾ cup nonfat milk
1 tbsp. wheat germ

Take cooked rice and place in bowl (after cooking rice according to package instructions). Top with honey and raisins to taste. Pour hot nonfat milk over ingredients. A great morning starter. *Variation:* Use as a dessert. ½ cup brown rice topped with honey or fructose.

This week covers _____ , _____ , _____ , to _____ , _____ , _____ .
month   day   year   month   day   year

Monday	E	Activity _____	Remarks (fitness): _____
	X	_____	_____
Resting Pulse Rate / **Weight At Rising**	E	Time _____	_____
	R	Distance _____	Remarks (personal): _____
	C	Pace _____	_____
	I	Effort: ☐ Easy ☐ Moderate	_____
	S E	☐ Hard ☐ Extreme	_____

Tuesday	E	Activity _____	Remarks (fitness): _____
	X	_____	_____
Resting Pulse Rate / **Weight At Rising**	E	Time _____	_____
	R	Distance _____	Remarks (personal): _____
	C	Pace _____	_____
	I	Effort: ☐ Easy ☐ Moderate	_____
	S E	☐ Hard ☐ Extreme	_____

Wednesday	E	Activity _____	Remarks (fitness): _____
	X	_____	_____
Resting Pulse Rate / **Weight At Rising**	E	Time _____	_____
	R	Distance _____	Remarks (personal): _____
	C	Pace _____	_____
	I	Effort: ☐ Easy ☐ Moderate	_____
	S E	☐ Hard ☐ Extreme	_____

Thursday	E	Activity _____	Remarks (fitness): _____
	X	_____	_____
Resting Pulse Rate / **Weight At Rising**	E	Time _____	_____
	R	Distance _____	Remarks (personal): _____
	C	Pace _____	_____
	I	Effort: ☐ Easy ☐ Moderate	_____
	S E	☐ Hard ☐ Extreme	_____

Friday	E	Activity _____	Remarks (fitness): _____
	X	_____	_____
Resting Pulse Rate / **Weight At Rising**	E	Time _____	_____
	R	Distance _____	Remarks (personal): _____
	C	Pace _____	_____
	I	Effort: ☐ Easy ☐ Moderate	_____
	S E	☐ Hard ☐ Extreme	_____

Saturday	E	Activity _____	Remarks (fitness): _____
	X	_____	_____
Resting Pulse Rate / **Weight At Rising**	E	Time _____	_____
	R	Distance _____	Remarks (personal): _____
	C	Pace _____	_____
	I	Effort: ☐ Easy ☐ Moderate	_____
	S E	☐ Hard ☐ Extreme	_____

Sunday	E	Activity _____	Remarks (fitness): _____
	X	_____	_____
Resting Pulse Rate / **Weight At Rising**	E	Time _____	_____
	R	Distance _____	Remarks (personal): _____
	C	Pace _____	_____
	I	Effort: ☐ Easy ☐ Moderate	_____
	S E	☐ Hard ☐ Extreme	_____

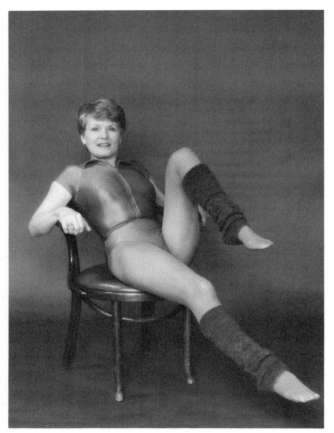

Knee into Chest
This exercise is mainly for those of you who are beginners and/or unable to bring both knees into your chest. Sit on edge of chair and try to lift right knee into your chest then left knee into your chest. Wonderful waist cincher.

Goals for this week:
1. _____
2. _____

Goals for this month:
1. _____
2. _____

Honey-Cheese Toast

¼ **cup cottage cheese**
1/8 tsp. cinnamon
1 tsp. honey

Mix above ingredients and spread on 100% whole wheat bread that has been toasted lightly and broil until spread is bubbly and golden brown.

Repeat this to yourself each morning: ''There are only three people who can get me fit: Me, myself and I.''

76

This week covers _____ , _____ , _____ , to _____ , _____ , _____ .
month　　　　day　　　　year　　　　　　month　　　　day　　　　year

Monday	E X E R C I S E	Activity _____ _____ Time _____ Distance _____ Pace _____ Effort: ☐ Easy　　☐ Moderate 　　　　☐ Hard　　☐ Extreme	Remarks (fitness): _____ _____ _____ Remarks (personal): _____ _____ _____
Resting Pulse Rate / **Weight At Rising**			

Tuesday	E X E R C I S E	Activity _____ _____ Time _____ Distance _____ Pace _____ Effort: ☐ Easy　　☐ Moderate 　　　　☐ Hard　　☐ Extreme	Remarks (fitness): _____ _____ _____ Remarks (personal): _____ _____ _____
Resting Pulse Rate / **Weight At Rising**			

Wednesday	E X E R C I S E	Activity _____ _____ Time _____ Distance _____ Pace _____ Effort: ☐ Easy　　☐ Moderate 　　　　☐ Hard　　☐ Extreme	Remarks (fitness): _____ _____ _____ Remarks (personal): _____ _____ _____
Resting Pulse Rate / **Weight At Rising**			

Thursday	E X E R C I S E	Activity _____ _____ Time _____ Distance _____ Pace _____ Effort: ☐ Easy　　☐ Moderate 　　　　☐ Hard　　☐ Extreme	Remarks (fitness): _____ _____ _____ Remarks (personal): _____ _____ _____
Resting Pulse Rate / **Weight At Rising**			

Friday	E X E R C I S E	Activity _____ _____ Time _____ Distance _____ Pace _____ Effort: ☐ Easy　　☐ Moderate 　　　　☐ Hard　　☐ Extreme	Remarks (fitness): _____ _____ _____ Remarks (personal): _____ _____ _____
Resting Pulse Rate / **Weight At Rising**			

Saturday	E X E R C I S E	Activity _____ _____ Time _____ Distance _____ Pace _____ Effort: ☐ Easy　　☐ Moderate 　　　　☐ Hard　　☐ Extreme	Remarks (fitness): _____ _____ _____ Remarks (personal): _____ _____ _____
Resting Pulse Rate / **Weight At Rising**			

Sunday	E X E R C I S E	Activity _____ _____ Time _____ Distance _____ Pace _____ Effort: ☐ Easy　　☐ Moderate 　　　　☐ Hard　　☐ Extreme	Remarks (fitness): _____ _____ _____ Remarks (personal): _____ _____ _____
Resting Pulse Rate / **Weight At Rising**			

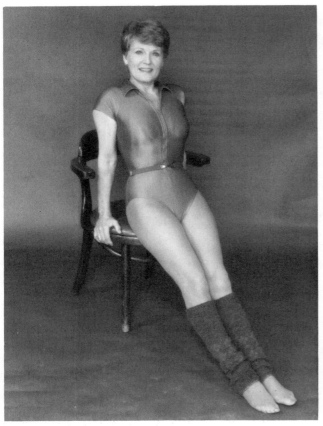

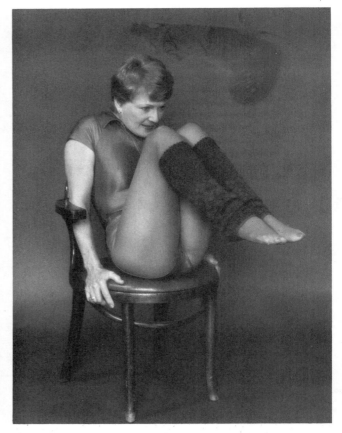

Knees into Chest

This exercise is excellent for the waist and helps strengthen the lower back. Using a solid, wide-based chair, sit on edge, your arms supporting yourself. Extend legs out, then in one smooth motion bring both knees in and try to touch your chest.

The only person who should not exercise to keep fit is the person who should have but didn't and found out too late; but his survivors should take the hint.

Goals for this week:

1. _____

2. _____

Goals for this month:

1. _____

2. _____

Lemon Scallops

Marinate 2 pounds of sea scallops in juice of 2 lemons with 4 cloves of finely chopped fresh garlic. Broil for approximately 3 minutes or until solid white. Season to taste and serve on a bed of watercress. Serves approximately five.

This week covers _____ , _____ , _____ , to _____ , _____ , _____ .
                    month   day   year   month   day   year

Monday	E	Activity _____	Remarks (fitness): _____
	X	_____	_____
Resting Pulse Rate	Weight At Rising	E R C	Time _____	_____
		I	Distance _____	Remarks (personal): _____
		S	Pace _____	_____
		E	Effort: ☐ Easy ☐ Moderate ☐ Hard ☐ Extreme	_____

Tuesday	E	Activity _____	Remarks (fitness): _____
	X	_____	_____
Resting Pulse Rate	Weight At Rising	E R C	Time _____	_____
		I	Distance _____	Remarks (personal): _____
		S	Pace _____	_____
		E	Effort: ☐ Easy ☐ Moderate ☐ Hard ☐ Extreme	_____

Wednesday	E	Activity _____	Remarks (fitness): _____
	X	_____	_____
Resting Pulse Rate	Weight At Rising	E R C	Time _____	_____
		I	Distance _____	Remarks (personal): _____
		S	Pace _____	_____
		E	Effort: ☐ Easy ☐ Moderate ☐ Hard ☐ Extreme	_____

Thursday	E	Activity _____	Remarks (fitness): _____
	X	_____	_____
Resting Pulse Rate	Weight At Rising	E R C	Time _____	_____
		I	Distance _____	Remarks (personal): _____
		S	Pace _____	_____
		E	Effort: ☐ Easy ☐ Moderate ☐ Hard ☐ Extreme	_____

Friday	E	Activity _____	Remarks (fitness): _____
	X	_____	_____
Resting Pulse Rate	Weight At Rising	E R C	Time _____	_____
		I	Distance _____	Remarks (personal): _____
		S	Pace _____	_____
		E	Effort: ☐ Easy ☐ Moderate ☐ Hard ☐ Extreme	_____

Saturday	E	Activity _____	Remarks (fitness): _____
	X	_____	_____
Resting Pulse Rate	Weight At Rising	E R C	Time _____	_____
		I	Distance _____	Remarks (personal): _____
		S	Pace _____	_____
		E	Effort: ☐ Easy ☐ Moderate ☐ Hard ☐ Extreme	_____

Sunday	E	Activity _____	Remarks (fitness): _____
	X	_____	_____
Resting Pulse Rate	Weight At Rising	E R C	Time _____	_____
		I	Distance _____	Remarks (personal): _____
		S	Pace _____	_____
		E	Effort: ☐ Easy ☐ Moderate ☐ Hard ☐ Extreme	_____

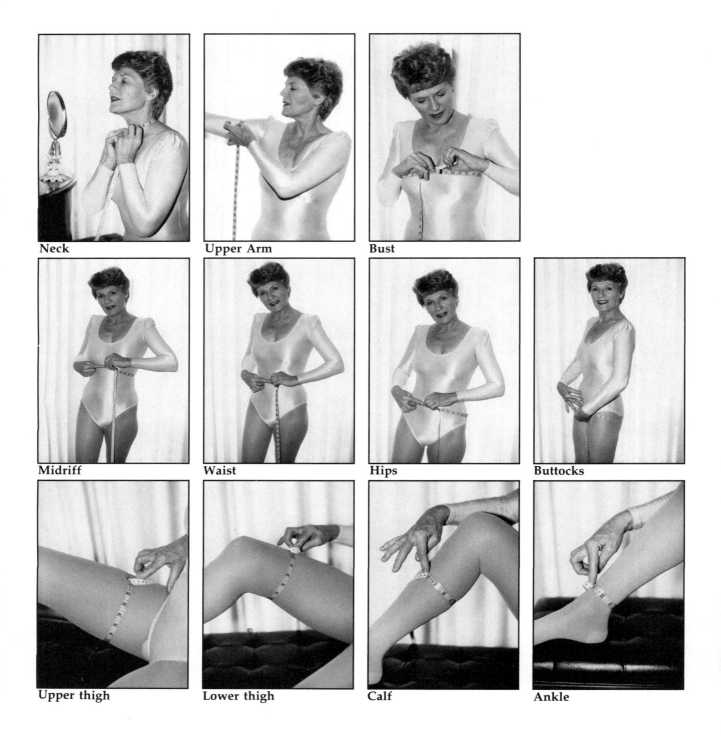

Neck

Upper Arm

Bust

Midriff

Waist

Hips

Buttocks

Upper thigh

Lower thigh

Calf

Ankle

Neck

Upper Arm

Bust

Midriff

Waist

Hips

Buttocks

Upper thigh

Lower thigh

Calf

Ankle

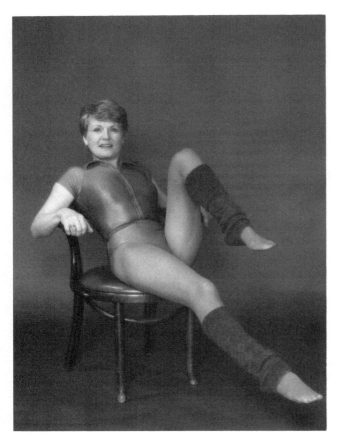

Bicycle
This is primarily the same exercise as the knee into the chest one seen on page 76; however, pump your legs as you would riding a bicycle. Another great exercise for the abdomen and upper thighs. Pump until tired, rest a few seconds and pump again.

A little fitness goes a long way. Ask any marathoner.

Goals for this week:
1. _____
2. _____

Goals for this month:
1. _____
2. _____

Wheat Pilaf

safflower oil
handful vermicelli noodles
1½ cups coarse wheat (bulgar)
14½ oz. can chicken broth or
   your chicken stock
1 cup water
2 cubes chicken or beef bouillon

In safflower oil, brown vermicelli noodles, stirring constantly so as not to burn. Keep stirring, then add wheat to vermicelli. Pour in broth, water and bouillon cubes and bring to a quick boil. Lower heat and simmer with cover until liquid is gone. Let set before serving.

This week covers _____ , _____ , _____ , to _____ , _____ , _____ .
month · day · year · month · day · year

Monday	E X E R C I S E	Activity _____ _____ Time _____ Distance _____ Pace _____ Effort: ☐ Easy ☐ Moderate ☐ Hard ☐ Extreme	Remarks (fitness): _____ _____ _____ Remarks (personal): _____ _____ _____
Resting Pulse Rate / **Weight At Rising**			

Tuesday	E X E R C I S E	Activity _____ _____ Time _____ Distance _____ Pace _____ Effort: ☐ Easy ☐ Moderate ☐ Hard ☐ Extreme	Remarks (fitness): _____ _____ _____ Remarks (personal): _____ _____ _____
Resting Pulse Rate / **Weight At Rising**			

Wednesday	E X E R C I S E	Activity _____ _____ Time _____ Distance _____ Pace _____ Effort: ☐ Easy ☐ Moderate ☐ Hard ☐ Extreme	Remarks (fitness): _____ _____ _____ Remarks (personal): _____ _____ _____
Resting Pulse Rate / **Weight At Rising**			

Thursday	E X E R C I S E	Activity _____ _____ Time _____ Distance _____ Pace _____ Effort: ☐ Easy ☐ Moderate ☐ Hard ☐ Extreme	Remarks (fitness): _____ _____ _____ Remarks (personal): _____ _____ _____
Resting Pulse Rate / **Weight At Rising**			

Friday	E X E R C I S E	Activity _____ _____ Time _____ Distance _____ Pace _____ Effort: ☐ Easy ☐ Moderate ☐ Hard ☐ Extreme	Remarks (fitness): _____ _____ _____ Remarks (personal): _____ _____ _____
Resting Pulse Rate / **Weight At Rising**			

Saturday	E X E R C I S E	Activity _____ _____ Time _____ Distance _____ Pace _____ Effort: ☐ Easy ☐ Moderate ☐ Hard ☐ Extreme	Remarks (fitness): _____ _____ _____ Remarks (personal): _____ _____ _____
Resting Pulse Rate / **Weight At Rising**			

Sunday	E X E R C I S E	Activity _____ _____ Time _____ Distance _____ Pace _____ Effort: ☐ Easy ☐ Moderate ☐ Hard ☐ Extreme	Remarks (fitness): _____ _____ _____ Remarks (personal): _____ _____ _____
Resting Pulse Rate / **Weight At Rising**			

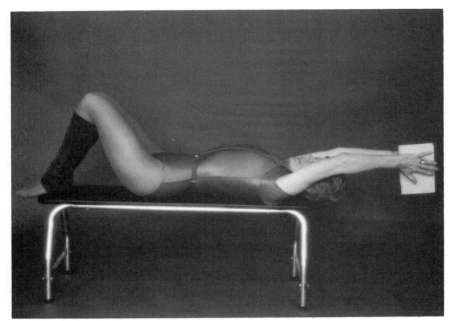

Pullovers

Wonderful exercise for posture, chest muscles and back of arms. Lie on bench or table. If you do not have a bench or table handy, a comfortable armless chair will suffice. Place a book between your hands. Keeping arms straight, let book pull your arms over as far as possible, then pull book over your chest.

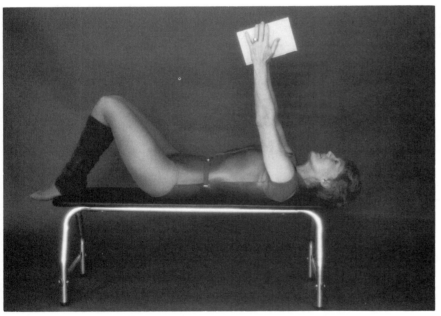

A day without exercise is merely a day.

Goals for this week:

1. _____

2. _____

Goals for this month:

1. _____

2. _____

Tomato Stuffed with Broccoli

1 tomato per person
cooked chopped broccoli
onion powder, garlic powder
grated cheese

Core tomato, stuff with cooked broccoli, onion and garlic powder, top with grated cheese. Place in baking dish under broiler and broil until ingredients are heated throughout.

This week covers _____ , _____ , _____ , to _____ , _____ , _____ .
                 month   day   year   month   day   year

Monday

Resting Pulse Rate	Weight At Rising

EXERCISE

Activity _____
_____
Time _____
Distance _____
Pace _____
Effort: ☐ Easy   ☐ Moderate
        ☐ Hard   ☐ Extreme

Remarks (fitness): _____
_____
_____
Remarks (personal): _____
_____
_____

Tuesday

Resting Pulse Rate	Weight At Rising

EXERCISE

Activity _____
_____
Time _____
Distance _____
Pace _____
Effort: ☐ Easy   ☐ Moderate
        ☐ Hard   ☐ Extreme

Remarks (fitness): _____
_____
_____
Remarks (personal): _____
_____
_____

Wednesday

Resting Pulse Rate	Weight At Rising

EXERCISE

Activity _____
_____
Time _____
Distance _____
Pace _____
Effort: ☐ Easy   ☐ Moderate
        ☐ Hard   ☐ Extreme

Remarks (fitness): _____
_____
_____
Remarks (personal): _____
_____
_____

Thursday

Resting Pulse Rate	Weight At Rising

EXERCISE

Activity _____
_____
Time _____
Distance _____
Pace _____
Effort: ☐ Easy   ☐ Moderate
        ☐ Hard   ☐ Extreme

Remarks (fitness): _____
_____
_____
Remarks (personal): _____
_____
_____

Friday

Resting Pulse Rate	Weight At Rising

EXERCISE

Activity _____
_____
Time _____
Distance _____
Pace _____
Effort: ☐ Easy   ☐ Moderate
        ☐ Hard   ☐ Extreme

Remarks (fitness): _____
_____
_____
Remarks (personal): _____
_____
_____

Saturday

Resting Pulse Rate	Weight At Rising

EXERCISE

Activity _____
_____
Time _____
Distance _____
Pace _____
Effort: ☐ Easy   ☐ Moderate
        ☐ Hard   ☐ Extreme

Remarks (fitness): _____
_____
_____
Remarks (personal): _____
_____
_____

Sunday

Resting Pulse Rate	Weight At Rising

EXERCISE

Activity _____
_____
Time _____
Distance _____
Pace _____
Effort: ☐ Easy   ☐ Moderate
        ☐ Hard   ☐ Extreme

Remarks (fitness): _____
_____
_____
Remarks (personal): _____
_____
_____

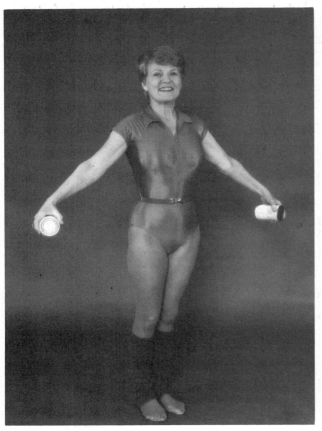 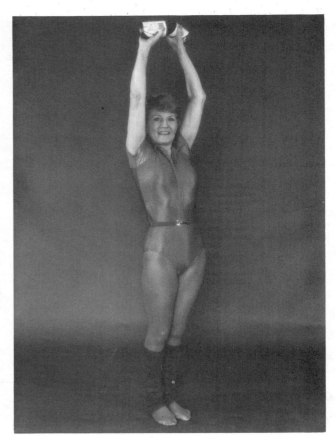

Lateral Raises
This exercise works the deltoid muscles (caps of the shoulders). Using some canned goods that you have on hand, stand erect and hold the two cans out from your sides. Keeping your arms straight, raise the cans over your head as pictured. Hold for a few seconds and then smoothly bring them back down. *Variation:* Books or weights can be used instead of cans.

**Fitness is a state of mind...
that affects your entire body.**

Goals for this week:
1. _____
2. _____

Goals for this month:
1. _____
2. _____

Broiled Eggplant Slices

1 eggplant
⅛ cup safflower oil
1 tbsp. garlic powder

Slice eggplant into ½-inch-thick slices. Place on cookie sheet lined with foil. Brush slices with safflower oil and sprinkle with garlic powder. Put under broiler until desired brownness and then turn slices over and follow same procedure.

This week covers _____ , _____ , _____ , **to** _____ , _____ , _____ .
month　　　　　day　　　　　year　　　　　　　　month　　　　　day　　　　　year

Monday	E X E R C I S E	Activity _____	Remarks (fitness): _____

Monday

Resting Pulse Rate	Weight At Rising

E X E R C I S E

Activity _____
_____
Time _____
Distance _____
Pace _____
Effort: ☐ Easy ☐ Moderate ☐ Hard ☐ Extreme

Remarks (fitness): _____
_____
_____
Remarks (personal): _____
_____
_____

Tuesday

Resting Pulse Rate	Weight At Rising

E X E R C I S E

Activity _____
_____
Time _____
Distance _____
Pace _____
Effort: ☐ Easy ☐ Moderate ☐ Hard ☐ Extreme

Remarks (fitness): _____
_____
_____
Remarks (personal): _____
_____
_____

Wednesday

Resting Pulse Rate	Weight At Rising

E X E R C I S E

Activity _____
_____
Time _____
Distance _____
Pace _____
Effort: ☐ Easy ☐ Moderate ☐ Hard ☐ Extreme

Remarks (fitness): _____
_____
_____
Remarks (personal): _____
_____
_____

Thursday

Resting Pulse Rate	Weight At Rising

E X E R C I S E

Activity _____
_____
Time _____
Distance _____
Pace _____
Effort: ☐ Easy ☐ Moderate ☐ Hard ☐ Extreme

Remarks (fitness): _____
_____
_____
Remarks (personal): _____
_____
_____

Friday

Resting Pulse Rate	Weight At Rising

E X E R C I S E

Activity _____
_____
Time _____
Distance _____
Pace _____
Effort: ☐ Easy ☐ Moderate ☐ Hard ☐ Extreme

Remarks (fitness): _____
_____
_____
Remarks (personal): _____
_____
_____

Saturday

Resting Pulse Rate	Weight At Rising

E X E R C I S E

Activity _____
_____
Time _____
Distance _____
Pace _____
Effort: ☐ Easy ☐ Moderate ☐ Hard ☐ Extreme

Remarks (fitness): _____
_____
_____
Remarks (personal): _____
_____
_____

Sunday

Resting Pulse Rate	Weight At Rising

E X E R C I S E

Activity _____
_____
Time _____
Distance _____
Pace _____
Effort: ☐ Easy ☐ Moderate ☐ Hard ☐ Extreme

Remarks (fitness): _____
_____
_____
Remarks (personal): _____
_____
_____

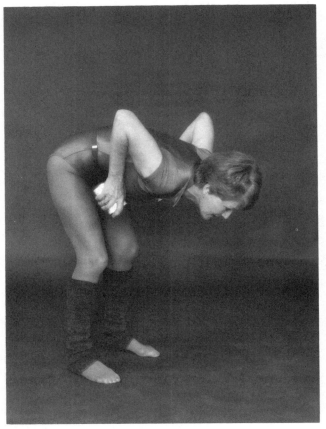

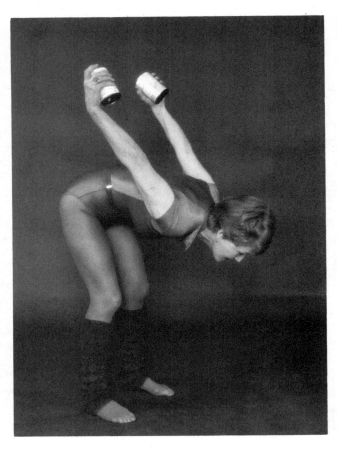

Arm Extensions
Helps tighten and tone the back of the upper arms. Bend over at waist, holding canned goods in both hands, feet shoulder-width apart, keeping elbows close to sides and as high as possible. Extend arms to the back with a smooth extension movement, trying to touch ceiling. This is basically the same exercise as seen on page 14; however it is more advanced in that you are using more weight (cans) which gives you more resistance. Books or weights may also be used.

Aerobic fitness gets to the heart of the matter.

Goals for this week:

1. _____

2. _____

Goals for this month:

1. _____

2. _____

Apple Delight

Grate 1 medium apple with skin. Add a squeeze of lemon and top with raisins and/or sunflower seeds. Top with honey (optional).

This week covers _____ , _____ , _____ , to _____ , _____ , _____ .
month · day · year · · month · day · year

Monday	E	

Monday

Resting Pulse Rate	Weight At Rising

E X E R C I S E

Activity _____
_____
Time _____
Distance _____
Pace _____
Effort: ☐ Easy ☐ Moderate
☐ Hard ☐ Extreme

Remarks (fitness): _____
_____
_____

Remarks (personal): _____
_____
_____

Tuesday

Resting Pulse Rate	Weight At Rising

E X E R C I S E

Activity _____
_____
Time _____
Distance _____
Pace _____
Effort: ☐ Easy ☐ Moderate
☐ Hard ☐ Extreme

Remarks (fitness): _____
_____
_____

Remarks (personal): _____
_____
_____

Wednesday

Resting Pulse Rate	Weight At Rising

E X E R C I S E

Activity _____
_____
Time _____
Distance _____
Pace _____
Effort: ☐ Easy ☐ Moderate
☐ Hard ☐ Extreme

Remarks (fitness): _____
_____
_____

Remarks (personal): _____
_____
_____

Thursday

Resting Pulse Rate	Weight At Rising

E X E R C I S E

Activity _____
_____
Time _____
Distance _____
Pace _____
Effort: ☐ Easy ☐ Moderate
☐ Hard ☐ Extreme

Remarks (fitness): _____
_____
_____

Remarks (personal): _____
_____
_____

Friday

Resting Pulse Rate	Weight At Rising

E X E R C I S E

Activity _____
_____
Time _____
Distance _____
Pace _____
Effort: ☐ Easy ☐ Moderate
☐ Hard ☐ Extreme

Remarks (fitness): _____
_____
_____

Remarks (personal): _____
_____
_____

Saturday

Resting Pulse Rate	Weight At Rising

E X E R C I S E

Activity _____
_____
Time _____
Distance _____
Pace _____
Effort: ☐ Easy ☐ Moderate
☐ Hard ☐ Extreme

Remarks (fitness): _____
_____
_____

Remarks (personal): _____
_____
_____

Sunday

Resting Pulse Rate	Weight At Rising

E X E R C I S E

Activity _____
_____
Time _____
Distance _____
Pace _____
Effort: ☐ Easy ☐ Moderate
☐ Hard ☐ Extreme

Remarks (fitness): _____
_____
_____

Remarks (personal): _____
_____
_____

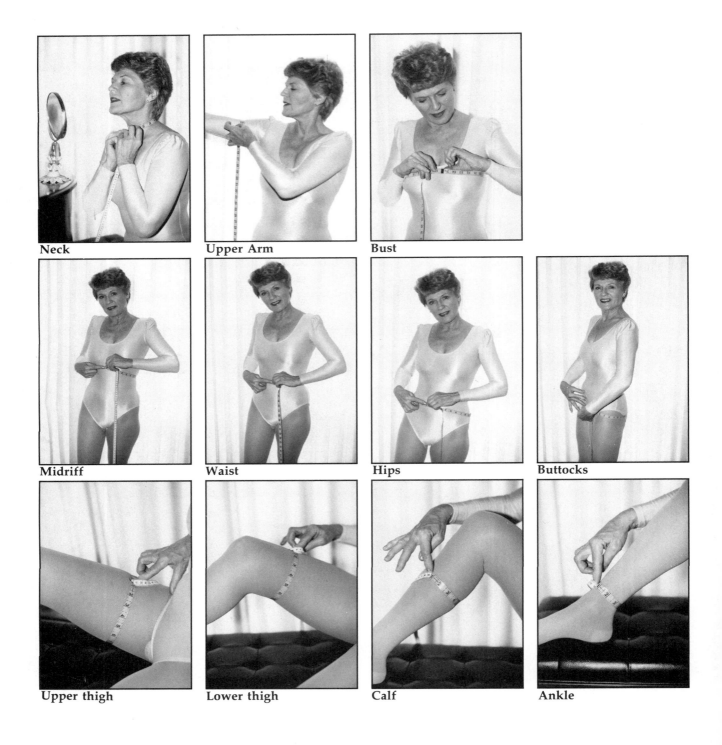

Neck

Upper Arm

Bust

Midriff

Waist

Hips

Buttocks

Upper thigh

Lower thigh

Calf

Ankle

Neck

Upper Arm

Bust

Midriff

Waist

Hips

Buttocks

Upper thigh

Lower thigh

Calf

Ankle

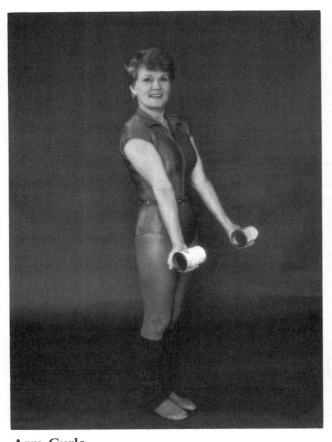

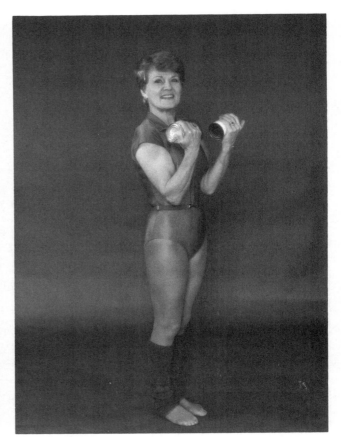

Arm Curls
Helps tone, tighten, and strengthen the
''belly'' of the forearm and front of the upper
arm. This is the basic curl used by weight-
lifters. Hold one 16-oz. can, heavy book or
weight in each hand with palms facing the
ceiling, arms tucked against your sides. Curl
lower arms from elbows (lower arm or
forearm is all that moves).

**If youth is wasted on the
young, why not recapture
your youth through fitness?**

Mock Sour Cream

1 cup lowfat cottage cheese
3-5 tbsp. nonfat powdered milk
2 tbsp. lemon juice
season to taste

Mix in blender to smooth texture.

Goals for this week:
1. _____
2. _____
Goals for this month:
1. _____
2. _____

This week covers _____ , _____ , _____ , to _____ , _____ , _____ .
month   day   year   month   day   year

Monday

Resting Pulse Rate	Weight At Rising

E X E R C I S E

Activity _____
_____
Time _____
Distance _____
Pace _____
Effort: ☐ Easy ☐ Moderate
☐ Hard ☐ Extreme

Remarks (fitness): _____
_____
Remarks (personal): _____
_____

Tuesday

Resting Pulse Rate	Weight At Rising

E X E R C I S E

Activity _____
_____
Time _____
Distance _____
Pace _____
Effort: ☐ Easy ☐ Moderate
☐ Hard ☐ Extreme

Remarks (fitness): _____
_____
Remarks (personal): _____
_____

Wednesday

Resting Pulse Rate	Weight At Rising

E X E R C I S E

Activity _____
_____
Time _____
Distance _____
Pace _____
Effort: ☐ Easy ☐ Moderate
☐ Hard ☐ Extreme

Remarks (fitness): _____
_____
Remarks (personal): _____
_____

Thursday

Resting Pulse Rate	Weight At Rising

E X E R C I S E

Activity _____
_____
Time _____
Distance _____
Pace _____
Effort: ☐ Easy ☐ Moderate
☐ Hard ☐ Extreme

Remarks (fitness): _____
_____
Remarks (personal): _____
_____

Friday

Resting Pulse Rate	Weight At Rising

E X E R C I S E

Activity _____
_____
Time _____
Distance _____
Pace _____
Effort: ☐ Easy ☐ Moderate
☐ Hard ☐ Extreme

Remarks (fitness): _____
_____
Remarks (personal): _____
_____

Saturday

Resting Pulse Rate	Weight At Rising

E X E R C I S E

Activity _____
_____
Time _____
Distance _____
Pace _____
Effort: ☐ Easy ☐ Moderate
☐ Hard ☐ Extreme

Remarks (fitness): _____
_____
Remarks (personal): _____
_____

Sunday

Resting Pulse Rate	Weight At Rising

E X E R C I S E

Activity _____
_____
Time _____
Distance _____
Pace _____
Effort: ☐ Easy ☐ Moderate
☐ Hard ☐ Extreme

Remarks (fitness): _____
_____
Remarks (personal): _____
_____

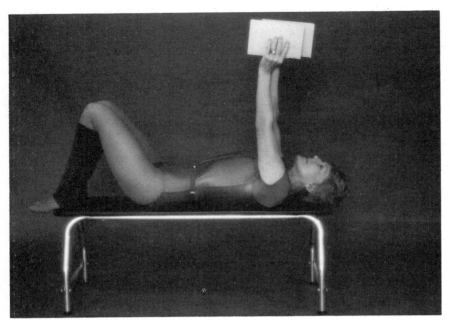

Supine Press
This is excellent for the back of arms and chest. Lie on your back, your knees up. Use two books. (As you get stronger, you can use larger, heavier books.) Hold the books up toward the ceiling. Then, bring them down smoothly to your shoulders. Hold for a second, and push them back up toward the ceiling. Repeat this one a dozen times. You can add more repeats as you get stronger.

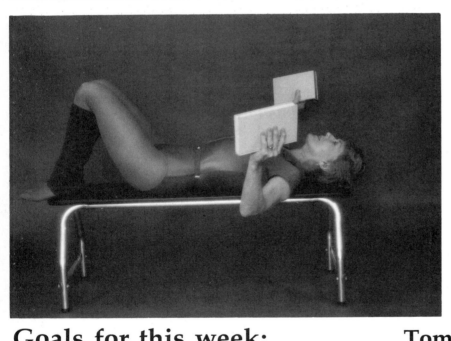

Inside everyone is a fit person waiting for the signal that it can free itself.

Goals for this week:

1. _____
2. _____

Goals for this month:

1. _____
2. _____

Tomato Yogurt Dip

½ **cup tomato sauce**
¼ **cup horseradish**
2 **tbsp. onion, minced**
½ **cup plain yogurt**

Mix tomato sauce, horseradish and onion. Fold in yogurt. Serve with assorted raw vegetables (cauliflower, broccoli, carrots, celery, jicama, etc.). Note: You may vary horseradish quantity according to taste.

This week covers _____ , _____ , _____ , to _____ , _____ , _____ .

      month   day   year   month   day   year

Monday

Resting Pulse Rate	Weight At Rising

EXERCISE

Activity _____
_____
Time _____
Distance _____
Pace _____
Effort: ☐ Easy ☐ Moderate
      ☐ Hard ☐ Extreme

Remarks (fitness): _____
_____
Remarks (personal): _____
_____

Tuesday

Resting Pulse Rate	Weight At Rising

EXERCISE

Activity _____
_____
Time _____
Distance _____
Pace _____
Effort: ☐ Easy ☐ Moderate
      ☐ Hard ☐ Extreme

Remarks (fitness): _____
_____
Remarks (personal): _____
_____

Wednesday

Resting Pulse Rate	Weight At Rising

EXERCISE

Activity _____
_____
Time _____
Distance _____
Pace _____
Effort: ☐ Easy ☐ Moderate
      ☐ Hard ☐ Extreme

Remarks (fitness): _____
_____
Remarks (personal): _____
_____

Thursday

Resting Pulse Rate	Weight At Rising

EXERCISE

Activity _____
_____
Time _____
Distance _____
Pace _____
Effort: ☐ Easy ☐ Moderate
      ☐ Hard ☐ Extreme

Remarks (fitness): _____
_____
Remarks (personal): _____
_____

Friday

Resting Pulse Rate	Weight At Rising

EXERCISE

Activity _____
_____
Time _____
Distance _____
Pace _____
Effort: ☐ Easy ☐ Moderate
      ☐ Hard ☐ Extreme

Remarks (fitness): _____
_____
Remarks (personal): _____
_____

Saturday

Resting Pulse Rate	Weight At Rising

EXERCISE

Activity _____
_____
Time _____
Distance _____
Pace _____
Effort: ☐ Easy ☐ Moderate
      ☐ Hard ☐ Extreme

Remarks (fitness): _____
_____
Remarks (personal): _____
_____

Sunday

Resting Pulse Rate	Weight At Rising

EXERCISE

Activity _____
Time _____
Distance _____
Pace _____
Effort: ☐ Easy ☐ Moderate
      ☐ Hard ☐ Extreme

Remarks (fitness): _____
_____
Remarks (personal): _____
_____

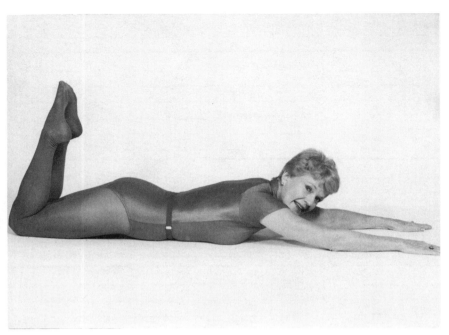

Leg Curls

This is an exercise that combines building muscles in the back of the legs and thighs with stretching. Lie on the floor, face down, bring your legs up from the knees. Reach out and stretch as far as you can. Hold for a count of five, lower your legs and release your stretch. Repeat as many times as is comfortable. Note: For more resistance, cross one foot on top of the other and curl legs.

Goals for this week:

1. _____
2. _____

Goals for this month:

1. _____
2. _____

Poached Pears or Apples

3 firm, ripe pears (use apples if
    pears aren't in season)
¾ cup honey
¾ cup water
1 tsp. lemon juice
1 tsp. vanilla extract

Core pears or apples and cut in half, leaving skins on. Combine honey, water, lemon juice and vanilla in saucepan, and bring to a boil. Add fruit, reduce heat and cook for approximately 20 minutes. Chill and serve with kiwi slices.

The nice thing about fitness is that if you work at it five days a week, you'll be fit all seven days that week.

This week covers _____ , _____ , _____ , to _____ , _____ , _____ .
month   day   year   month   day   year

Monday

Resting Pulse Rate	Weight At Rising

EXERCISE

Activity _____
_____
Time _____
Distance _____
Pace _____
Effort: ☐ Easy   ☐ Moderate
         ☐ Hard   ☐ Extreme

Remarks (fitness): _____
_____
_____
Remarks (personal): _____
_____
_____

Tuesday

Resting Pulse Rate	Weight At Rising

EXERCISE

Activity _____
_____
Time _____
Distance _____
Pace _____
Effort: ☐ Easy   ☐ Moderate
         ☐ Hard   ☐ Extreme

Remarks (fitness): _____
_____
_____
Remarks (personal): _____
_____
_____

Wednesday

Resting Pulse Rate	Weight At Rising

EXERCISE

Activity _____
_____
Time _____
Distance _____
Pace _____
Effort: ☐ Easy   ☐ Moderate
         ☐ Hard   ☐ Extreme

Remarks (fitness): _____
_____
_____
Remarks (personal): _____
_____
_____

Thursday

Resting Pulse Rate	Weight At Rising

EXERCISE

Activity _____
_____
Time _____
Distance _____
Pace _____
Effort: ☐ Easy   ☐ Moderate
         ☐ Hard   ☐ Extreme

Remarks (fitness): _____
_____
_____
Remarks (personal): _____
_____
_____

Friday

Resting Pulse Rate	Weight At Rising

EXERCISE

Activity _____
_____
Time _____
Distance _____
Pace _____
Effort: ☐ Easy   ☐ Moderate
         ☐ Hard   ☐ Extreme

Remarks (fitness): _____
_____
_____
Remarks (personal): _____
_____
_____

Saturday

Resting Pulse Rate	Weight At Rising

EXERCISE

Activity _____
_____
Time _____
Distance _____
Pace _____
Effort: ☐ Easy   ☐ Moderate
         ☐ Hard   ☐ Extreme

Remarks (fitness): _____
_____
_____
Remarks (personal): _____
_____
_____

Sunday

Resting Pulse Rate	Weight At Rising

EXERCISE

Activity _____
_____
Time _____
Distance _____
Pace _____
Effort: ☐ Easy   ☐ Moderate
         ☐ Hard   ☐ Extreme

Remarks (fitness): _____
_____
_____
Remarks (personal): _____
_____
_____

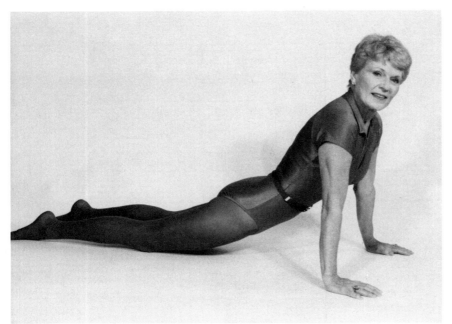

Cobra Stretch
A great stretch! Spread your lower body out comfortably on the floor and lift your upper body with your arms. Arch your back, head up, stretch, hold for five seconds, release and repeat.

Goals for this week:

1. _____

2. _____

Goals for this month:

1. _____

2. _____

Think positively about yourself, and you'll have to do positive things for yourself.

Cabbage and Tofu

½ head cabbage, cut into
   large pieces
1 green pepper, chopped
1 cup bean sprouts
2 slices tofu (¾- to 1-inch), cubed
greens (add anything you like, such
   as collards, swiss chard, etc.)
season to taste

Sauté above ingredients together lightly and serve.

This week covers _____ , _____ , _____ , to _____ , _____ , _____ .
month   day   year   month   day   year

Monday	E X E R C I S E	Activity _____ _____ Time _____ Distance _____ Pace _____ Effort: ☐ Easy ☐ Moderate ☐ Hard ☐ Extreme	Remarks (fitness): _____ _____ _____ Remarks (personal): _____ _____ _____
Resting Pulse Rate | **Weight At Rising**			

Tuesday	E X E R C I S E	Activity _____ _____ Time _____ Distance _____ Pace _____ Effort: ☐ Easy ☐ Moderate ☐ Hard ☐ Extreme	Remarks (fitness): _____ _____ _____ Remarks (personal): _____ _____ _____
Resting Pulse Rate | **Weight At Rising**			

Wednesday	E X E R C I S E	Activity _____ _____ Time _____ Distance _____ Pace _____ Effort: ☐ Easy ☐ Moderate ☐ Hard ☐ Extreme	Remarks (fitness): _____ _____ _____ Remarks (personal): _____ _____ _____
Resting Pulse Rate | **Weight At Rising**			

Thursday	E X E R C I S E	Activity _____ _____ Time _____ Distance _____ Pace _____ Effort: ☐ Easy ☐ Moderate ☐ Hard ☐ Extreme	Remarks (fitness): _____ _____ _____ Remarks (personal): _____ _____ _____
Resting Pulse Rate | **Weight At Rising**			

Friday	E X E R C I S E	Activity _____ _____ Time _____ Distance _____ Pace _____ Effort: ☐ Easy ☐ Moderate ☐ Hard ☐ Extreme	Remarks (fitness): _____ _____ _____ Remarks (personal): _____ _____ _____
Resting Pulse Rate | **Weight At Rising**			

Saturday	E X E R C I S E	Activity _____ _____ Time _____ Distance _____ Pace _____ Effort: ☐ Easy ☐ Moderate ☐ Hard ☐ Extreme	Remarks (fitness): _____ _____ _____ Remarks (personal): _____ _____ _____
Resting Pulse Rate | **Weight At Rising**			

Sunday	E X E R C I S E	Activity _____ _____ Time _____ Distance _____ Pace _____ Effort: ☐ Easy ☐ Moderate ☐ Hard ☐ Extreme	Remarks (fitness): _____ _____ _____ Remarks (personal): _____ _____ _____
Resting Pulse Rate | **Weight At Rising**			

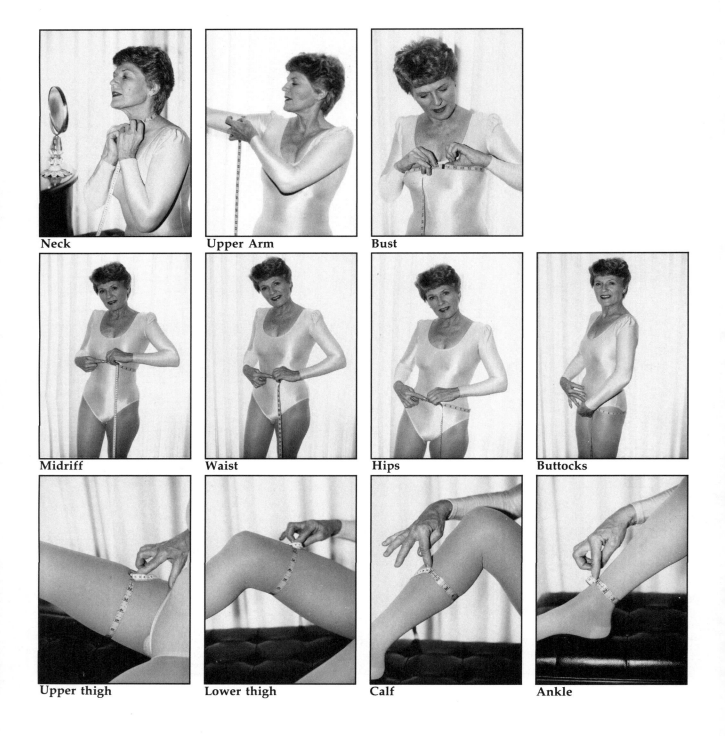

Neck

Upper Arm

Bust

Midriff

Waist

Hips

Buttocks

Upper thigh

Lower thigh

Calf

Ankle

Neck

Upper Arm

Bust

Midriff

Waist

Hips

Buttocks

Upper thigh

Lower thigh

Calf

Ankle

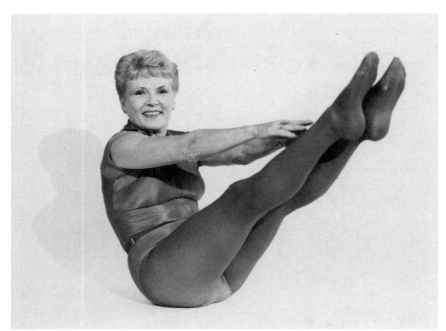

Jack Knife
Advanced exercise for the front of the midsection. Extend hands behind head. Lift legs and body simultaneously. Try to touch toes with your hands. Start with one or two and work up to 20. This is difficult at first; however, with practice you can make it.

Goals for this week:
1. _____
2. _____

Goals for this month:
1. _____
2. _____

A day without sunshine is a perfect day to exercise inside.

High-Protein Pancakes
4 eggs
1 cup cottage cheese
2 tbsp. safflower oil
½ cup oatmeal (or ¼ cup wheat germ & ¼ cup oatmeal)
¼ tsp. salt
Place all ingredients in a blender and mix thoroughly. Drop by tablespoon onto hot greased frying pan or griddle. Serves 3-4. *Variation:* ½ cup whole wheat flour may also be used instead of oatmeal.

This week covers _____ , _____ , _____ , to _____ , _____ , _____ .
                month   day   year   month   day   year

Monday

Resting Pulse Rate	Weight At Rising

EXERCISE

Activity _____
_____
Time _____
Distance _____
Pace _____
Effort: ☐ Easy   ☐ Moderate   ☐ Hard   ☐ Extreme

Remarks (fitness): _____
_____
Remarks (personal): _____
_____
_____

Tuesday

Resting Pulse Rate	Weight At Rising

EXERCISE

Activity _____
_____
Time _____
Distance _____
Pace _____
Effort: ☐ Easy   ☐ Moderate   ☐ Hard   ☐ Extreme

Remarks (fitness): _____
_____
Remarks (personal): _____
_____
_____

Wednesday

Resting Pulse Rate	Weight At Rising

EXERCISE

Activity _____
_____
Time _____
Distance _____
Pace _____
Effort: ☐ Easy   ☐ Moderate   ☐ Hard   ☐ Extreme

Remarks (fitness): _____
_____
Remarks (personal): _____
_____
_____

Thursday

Resting Pulse Rate	Weight At Rising

EXERCISE

Activity _____
_____
Time _____
Distance _____
Pace _____
Effort: ☐ Easy   ☐ Moderate   ☐ Hard   ☐ Extreme

Remarks (fitness): _____
_____
Remarks (personal): _____
_____
_____

Friday

Resting Pulse Rate	Weight At Rising

EXERCISE

Activity _____
_____
Time _____
Distance _____
Pace _____
Effort: ☐ Easy   ☐ Moderate   ☐ Hard   ☐ Extreme

Remarks (fitness): _____
_____
Remarks (personal): _____
_____
_____

Saturday

Resting Pulse Rate	Weight At Rising

EXERCISE

Activity _____
_____
Time _____
Distance _____
Pace _____
Effort: ☐ Easy   ☐ Moderate   ☐ Hard   ☐ Extreme

Remarks (fitness): _____
_____
Remarks (personal): _____
_____
_____

Sunday

Resting Pulse Rate	Weight At Rising

EXERCISE

Activity _____
_____
Time _____
Distance _____
Pace _____
Effort: ☐ Easy   ☐ Moderate   ☐ Hard   ☐ Extreme

Remarks (fitness): _____
_____
Remarks (personal): _____
_____

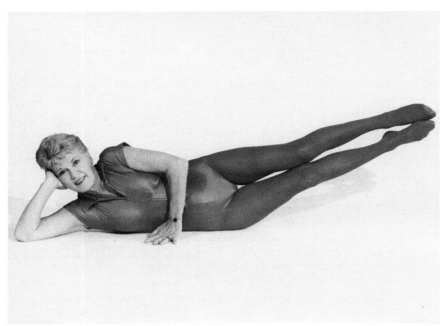

Hips and Thighs

This one is terrific for the hips and inner thighs. Lie on the floor, on your side, using your lower arm to support your head. Now, raise your upper leg, keeping it straight. Then, a second later, bring your lower leg up to meet it, keeping it straight. Hold for two seconds, then lower the lower leg, and then lower the upper leg after it. Pause for two seconds and repeat. Then turn over and do it on the other side.

The sickest person is the one who sits around waiting to get sick.

Blender Soup

1 can chicken broth or homemade chicken stock
1 carrot, chopped
½ zucchini, chopped
1 small bell pepper, chopped
1 stalk celery, chopped

Mix the above ingredients in blender. Pour in saucepan and bring to boil. (Note: You may substitute any of the vegetables mentioned for the ones you have sitting in your refrigerator waiting to be used.) Serves 2 or 3.

Variation:
1 cup water
1 can chicken broth
¾ cup each of celery, bell pepper, potato, cauliflower, carrots, cucumber, zucchini (all chopped)

Heat and serve.

Goals for this week:
1. _____
2. _____

Goals for this month:
1. _____
2. _____

This week covers _____ , _____ , _____ , to _____ , _____ , _____ .
month   day   year   month   day   year

Monday	E X E R C I S E	Activity _____

Monday

Monday

Resting Pulse Rate | Weight At Rising

EXERCISE

Activity _____
_____
Time _____
Distance _____
Pace _____
Effort: ☐ Easy ☐ Moderate ☐ Hard ☐ Extreme

Remarks (fitness): _____
_____
_____
Remarks (personal): _____
_____
_____

Tuesday

Tuesday

Resting Pulse Rate | Weight At Rising

EXERCISE

Activity _____
_____
Time _____
Distance _____
Pace _____
Effort: ☐ Easy ☐ Moderate ☐ Hard ☐ Extreme

Remarks (fitness): _____
_____
_____
Remarks (personal): _____
_____
_____

Wednesday

Wednesday

Resting Pulse Rate | Weight At Rising

EXERCISE

Activity _____
_____
Time _____
Distance _____
Pace _____
Effort: ☐ Easy ☐ Moderate ☐ Hard ☐ Extreme

Remarks (fitness): _____
_____
_____
Remarks (personal): _____
_____
_____

Thursday

Thursday

Resting Pulse Rate | Weight At Rising

EXERCISE

Activity _____
_____
Time _____
Distance _____
Pace _____
Effort: ☐ Easy ☐ Moderate ☐ Hard ☐ Extreme

Remarks (fitness): _____
_____
_____
Remarks (personal): _____
_____
_____

Friday

Friday

Resting Pulse Rate | Weight At Rising

EXERCISE

Activity _____
_____
Time _____
Distance _____
Pace _____
Effort: ☐ Easy ☐ Moderate ☐ Hard ☐ Extreme

Remarks (fitness): _____
_____
_____
Remarks (personal): _____
_____
_____

Saturday

Saturday

Resting Pulse Rate | Weight At Rising

EXERCISE

Activity _____
_____
Time _____
Distance _____
Pace _____
Effort: ☐ Easy ☐ Moderate ☐ Hard ☐ Extreme

Remarks (fitness): _____
_____
_____
Remarks (personal): _____
_____
_____

Sunday

Sunday

Resting Pulse Rate | Weight At Rising

EXERCISE

Activity _____
_____
Time _____
Distance _____
Pace _____
Effort: ☐ Easy ☐ Moderate ☐ Hard ☐ Extreme

Remarks (fitness): _____
_____
_____
Remarks (personal): _____
_____
_____

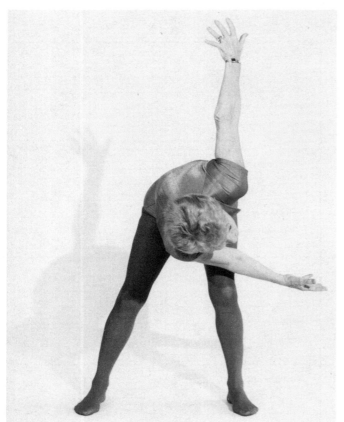

Windmills

This exercise is great for the sides of the waist and the backs of the arms. Bend over at the waist, arms stretched out; simultaneously swing your right arm across your body and try to touch your left hand to the ceiling; then swing back your left arm and extend the right hand to the ceiling. Do this one as rapidly as possible.

Beware! Fitness is addictive. And contagious.

Goals for this week:

1. _____

2. _____

Goals for this month:

1. _____

2. _____

Yogurt-Banana Freeze

2 cups very ripe bananas
1½ cups plain yogurt

Put in blender and mix well. Pour into ice cube trays and freeze. Before serving, put pieces through blender again. (This will make it appear like soft ice cream or frozen yogurt.) *Variations:* Add pineapple (fresh or canned) to mixture in blender after freezing. You may use any fruit desired; however, pineapple will give a sweeter flavor. You may also add apple, orange, or pineapple juices. Experiment with this one; be creative.

This week covers _____ , _____ , _____ , to _____ , _____ , _____ .
month   day   year   month   day   year

| Monday | E X E R C I S E | Activity _____ | Remarks (fitness): _____ |
| Resting Pulse Rate / Weight At Rising | | _____
Time _____
Distance _____
Pace _____
Effort: ☐ Easy ☐ Moderate
☐ Hard ☐ Extreme | Remarks (personal): _____ |

| Tuesday | E X E R C I S E | Activity _____ | Remarks (fitness): _____ |
| Resting Pulse Rate / Weight At Rising | | _____
Time _____
Distance _____
Pace _____
Effort: ☐ Easy ☐ Moderate
☐ Hard ☐ Extreme | Remarks (personal): _____ |

| Wednesday | E X E R C I S E | Activity _____ | Remarks (fitness): _____ |
| Resting Pulse Rate / Weight At Rising | | _____
Time _____
Distance _____
Pace _____
Effort: ☐ Easy ☐ Moderate
☐ Hard ☐ Extreme | Remarks (personal): _____ |

| Thursday | E X E R C I S E | Activity _____ | Remarks (fitness): _____ |
| Resting Pulse Rate / Weight At Rising | | _____
Time _____
Distance _____
Pace _____
Effort: ☐ Easy ☐ Moderate
☐ Hard ☐ Extreme | Remarks (personal): _____ |

| Friday | E X E R C I S E | Activity _____ | Remarks (fitness): _____ |
| Resting Pulse Rate / Weight At Rising | | _____
Time _____
Distance _____
Pace _____
Effort: ☐ Easy ☐ Moderate
☐ Hard ☐ Extreme | Remarks (personal): _____ |

| Saturday | E X E R C I S E | Activity _____ | Remarks (fitness): _____ |
| Resting Pulse Rate / Weight At Rising | | _____
Time _____
Distance _____
Pace _____
Effort: ☐ Easy ☐ Moderate
☐ Hard ☐ Extreme | Remarks (personal): _____ |

| Sunday | E X E R C I S E | Activity _____ | Remarks (fitness): _____ |
| Resting Pulse Rate / Weight At Rising | | _____
Time _____
Distance _____
Pace _____
Effort: ☐ Easy ☐ Moderate
☐ Hard ☐ Extreme | Remarks (personal): _____ |

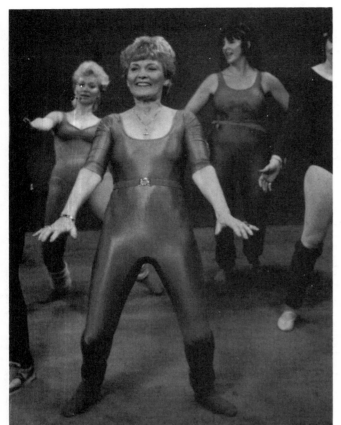

To get ahead in the arms race, do a dozen push-ups today.

Goals for this week:
1. _____
2. _____

Goals for this month:
1. _____
2. _____

Comfort while Exercising
One other matter that I'd like to mention while I have the opportunity is that when you exercise, you should be as comfortable as possible. I like to wear a one-piece suit because it allows me to move freely. There are many, many fashions on the market that will work beautifully for you. Or, if you want to keep it simple, pull out an old sweatshirt and go to it.

Dilled Peppers and Cukes
red pepper rings
scored sliced cucumbers
Arrange pepper rings and cucumbers on bed of watercress. Top with Dill Dressing.
Dill Dressing:
1 tbsp. mayonnaise
1 tbsp. yogurt (plain)
dill weed to taste
Mix all ingredients and serve.

This week covers _____ , _____ , _____ , to _____ , _____ , _____ .
                  month   day   year   month   day   year

Monday

Resting Pulse Rate	Weight At Rising

EXERCISE

Activity _____
_____
Time _____
Distance _____
Pace _____
Effort: ☐ Easy ☐ Moderate ☐ Hard ☐ Extreme

Remarks (fitness): _____
_____

Remarks (personal): _____
_____
_____

Tuesday

Resting Pulse Rate	Weight At Rising

EXERCISE

Activity _____
_____
Time _____
Distance _____
Pace _____
Effort: ☐ Easy ☐ Moderate ☐ Hard ☐ Extreme

Remarks (fitness): _____
_____

Remarks (personal): _____
_____
_____

Wednesday

Resting Pulse Rate	Weight At Rising

EXERCISE

Activity _____
_____
Time _____
Distance _____
Pace _____
Effort: ☐ Easy ☐ Moderate ☐ Hard ☐ Extreme

Remarks (fitness): _____
_____

Remarks (personal): _____
_____
_____

Thursday

Resting Pulse Rate	Weight At Rising

EXERCISE

Activity _____
_____
Time _____
Distance _____
Pace _____
Effort: ☐ Easy ☐ Moderate ☐ Hard ☐ Extreme

Remarks (fitness): _____
_____

Remarks (personal): _____
_____
_____

Friday

Resting Pulse Rate	Weight At Rising

EXERCISE

Activity _____
_____
Time _____
Distance _____
Pace _____
Effort: ☐ Easy ☐ Moderate ☐ Hard ☐ Extreme

Remarks (fitness): _____
_____

Remarks (personal): _____
_____
_____

Saturday

Resting Pulse Rate	Weight At Rising

EXERCISE

Activity _____
_____
Time _____
Distance _____
Pace _____
Effort: ☐ Easy ☐ Moderate ☐ Hard ☐ Extreme

Remarks (fitness): _____
_____

Remarks (personal): _____
_____
_____

Sunday

Resting Pulse Rate	Weight At Rising

EXERCISE

Activity _____
_____
Time _____
Distance _____
Pace _____
Effort: ☐ Easy ☐ Moderate ☐ Hard ☐ Extreme

Remarks (fitness): _____
_____

Remarks (personal): _____
_____
_____

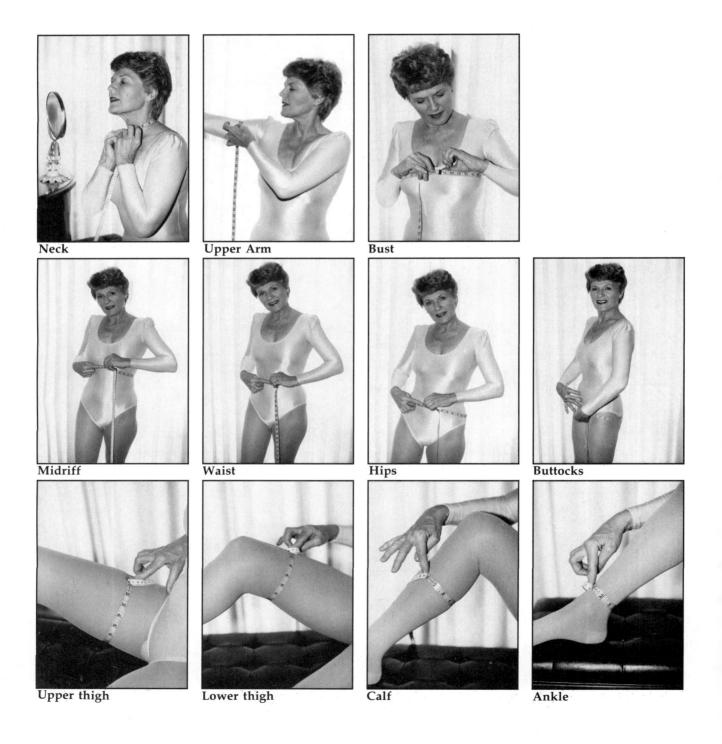

Neck

Upper Arm

Bust

Midriff

Waist

Hips

Buttocks

Upper thigh

Lower thigh

Calf

Ankle

Neck

Upper Arm

Bust

Midriff

Waist

Hips

Buttocks

Upper thigh

Lower thigh

Calf

Ankle

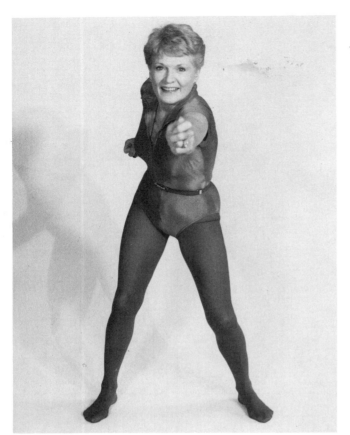

The way to a man's—or woman's—heart is through aerobic exercise.

Goals for this week:

1. _____
2. _____

Goals for this month:

1. _____
2. _____

Punching

If done correctly, this exercise affects most of the body's muscles. It is also wonderful for cardiovascular conditioning. Bend slightly at the knees. Pretend you are hitting a punching bag. Attempt to hit the wall behind you with your elbows on the back swings of your arms; then punch out, trying to hit the wall in front of you. Do not be surprised if at first this exercise proves to be quite exhausting.

Jon LaLanne's Quick Lunch

lettuce
drained sardines or water pack tuna
tomato slices
2 heaping tbsp. cottage cheese
whole wheat crackers

On a bed of lettuce, arrange sardines or tuna with tomato slices. Top with cottage cheese, and serve with whole wheat crackers.

This week covers _____ , _____ , _____ , to _____ , _____ , _____ .
month   day   year   month   day   year

Monday	E X E R C I S E	Activity _____ _____ Time _____ Distance _____ Pace _____ Effort: ☐ Easy ☐ Moderate ☐ Hard ☐ Extreme	Remarks (fitness): _____ _____ _____ Remarks (personal): _____ _____ _____
Resting Pulse Rate / **Weight At Rising**			

Tuesday	E X E R C I S E	Activity _____ _____ Time _____ Distance _____ Pace _____ Effort: ☐ Easy ☐ Moderate ☐ Hard ☐ Extreme	Remarks (fitness): _____ _____ _____ Remarks (personal): _____ _____ _____
Resting Pulse Rate / **Weight At Rising**			

Wednesday	E X E R C I S E	Activity _____ _____ Time _____ Distance _____ Pace _____ Effort: ☐ Easy ☐ Moderate ☐ Hard ☐ Extreme	Remarks (fitness): _____ _____ _____ Remarks (personal): _____ _____ _____
Resting Pulse Rate / **Weight At Rising**			

Thursday	E X E R C I S E	Activity _____ _____ Time _____ Distance _____ Pace _____ Effort: ☐ Easy ☐ Moderate ☐ Hard ☐ Extreme	Remarks (fitness): _____ _____ _____ Remarks (personal): _____ _____ _____
Resting Pulse Rate / **Weight At Rising**			

Friday	E X E R C I S E	Activity _____ _____ Time _____ Distance _____ Pace _____ Effort: ☐ Easy ☐ Moderate ☐ Hard ☐ Extreme	Remarks (fitness): _____ _____ _____ Remarks (personal): _____ _____ _____
Resting Pulse Rate / **Weight At Rising**			

Saturday	E X E R C I S E	Activity _____ _____ Time _____ Distance _____ Pace _____ Effort: ☐ Easy ☐ Moderate ☐ Hard ☐ Extreme	Remarks (fitness): _____ _____ _____ Remarks (personal): _____ _____ _____
Resting Pulse Rate / **Weight At Rising**			

Sunday	E X E R C I S E	Activity _____ _____ Time _____ Distance _____ Pace _____ Effort: ☐ Easy ☐ Moderate ☐ Hard ☐ Extreme	Remarks (fitness): _____ _____ _____ Remarks (personal): _____ _____ _____
Resting Pulse Rate / **Weight At Rising**			

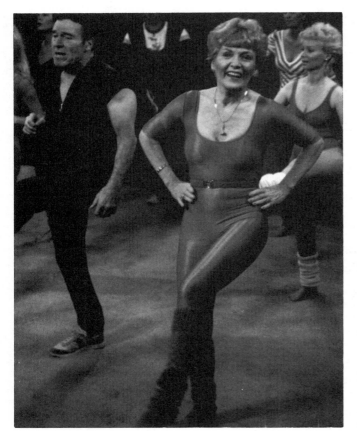

Invest in your well-being. Sell yourself on fitness.

Goals for this week:
1. _____
2. _____

Goals for this month:
1. _____
2. _____

You Got Rhythm

I like to do my exercises by getting into a rhythm. You can tell from this picture that the music is perfect, and that we're all getting into the rhythm. Unfortunately, the camera, which never lies, has caught Jack singing. Now Jack's an inspiration when he exercises, but if you've ever heard him sing... he's fantastic!

Date and Nut Squares

2 eggs
⅓ cup honey
½ tsp. vanilla
½ cup flour
½ tsp. baking powder
1 cup walnuts, chopped
2 cups dates, finely chopped

Beat eggs until foamy. Beat in honey and vanilla. Mix in remaining ingredients. Put into an oiled and floured 8-inch square pan and bake at 375 degrees for approximately 25-30 minutes, or until top has dull crust. Cut into squares and cool. Remove from pan. Makes 12 squares.

This week covers _____ , _____ , _____ , to _____ , _____ , _____ .
month   day   year   month   day   year

Monday

Resting Pulse Rate	Weight At Rising

EXERCISE

Activity _____
_____
Time _____
Distance _____
Pace _____
Effort: ☐ Easy   ☐ Moderate
       ☐ Hard   ☐ Extreme

Remarks (fitness): _____
_____
_____

Remarks (personal): _____
_____
_____

Tuesday

Resting Pulse Rate	Weight At Rising

EXERCISE

Activity _____
_____
Time _____
Distance _____
Pace _____
Effort: ☐ Easy   ☐ Moderate
       ☐ Hard   ☐ Extreme

Remarks (fitness): _____
_____
_____

Remarks (personal): _____
_____
_____

Wednesday

Resting Pulse Rate	Weight At Rising

EXERCISE

Activity _____
_____
Time _____
Distance _____
Pace _____
Effort: ☐ Easy   ☐ Moderate
       ☐ Hard   ☐ Extreme

Remarks (fitness): _____
_____
_____

Remarks (personal): _____
_____
_____

Thursday

Resting Pulse Rate	Weight At Rising

EXERCISE

Activity _____
_____
Time _____
Distance _____
Pace _____
Effort: ☐ Easy   ☐ Moderate
       ☐ Hard   ☐ Extreme

Remarks (fitness): _____
_____
_____

Remarks (personal): _____
_____
_____

Friday

Resting Pulse Rate	Weight At Rising

EXERCISE

Activity _____
_____
Time _____
Distance _____
Pace _____
Effort: ☐ Easy   ☐ Moderate
       ☐ Hard   ☐ Extreme

Remarks (fitness): _____
_____
_____

Remarks (personal): _____
_____
_____

Saturday

Resting Pulse Rate	Weight At Rising

EXERCISE

Activity _____
_____
Time _____
Distance _____
Pace _____
Effort: ☐ Easy   ☐ Moderate
       ☐ Hard   ☐ Extreme

Remarks (fitness): _____
_____
_____

Remarks (personal): _____
_____
_____

Sunday

Resting Pulse Rate	Weight At Rising

EXERCISE

Activity _____
_____
Time _____
Distance _____
Pace _____
Effort: ☐ Easy   ☐ Moderate
       ☐ Hard   ☐ Extreme

Remarks (fitness): _____
_____
_____

Remarks (personal): _____
_____
_____

One push-up is worth a dozen excuses.

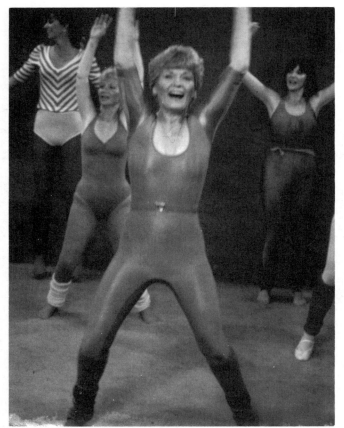

Let the Fun Shine Through
When you really get into your exercises, when you let your stretch go wild, when you get into the rhythm, when you begin to love the movement of your own body, if it happens to make you happy, don't hesitate to allow a smile to cross your face. It is only a reflection of how happy your body is to be doing what it does best—moving.

Goals for this week:
1. _____
2. _____

Goals for this month:
1. _____
2. _____

Wheat-Soya Spaghetti

2 cups cooked wheat-soya spaghetti
1 6½-oz. portion of chopped clams and/or shrimp or scallops
½ cup chopped tomatoes (preferably fresh

In a frying pan, mix above together until desired warmth. Season to taste. *Variation:* Add mushrooms and grated carrot.

This week covers _____ , _____ , _____ , to _____ , _____ , _____ .
month   day   year   month   day   year

Monday	E X E R C I S E	Activity _____ _____ Time _____ Distance _____ Pace _____ Effort: ☐ Easy ☐ Moderate ☐ Hard ☐ Extreme	Remarks (fitness): _____ _____ _____ Remarks (personal): _____ _____ _____
Resting Pulse Rate / **Weight At Rising**			

Tuesday	E X E R C I S E	Activity _____ _____ Time _____ Distance _____ Pace _____ Effort: ☐ Easy ☐ Moderate ☐ Hard ☐ Extreme	Remarks (fitness): _____ _____ _____ Remarks (personal): _____ _____ _____
Resting Pulse Rate / **Weight At Rising**			

Wednesday	E X E R C I S E	Activity _____ _____ Time _____ Distance _____ Pace _____ Effort: ☐ Easy ☐ Moderate ☐ Hard ☐ Extreme	Remarks (fitness): _____ _____ _____ Remarks (personal): _____ _____ _____
Resting Pulse Rate / **Weight At Rising**			

Thursday	E X E R C I S E	Activity _____ _____ Time _____ Distance _____ Pace _____ Effort: ☐ Easy ☐ Moderate ☐ Hard ☐ Extreme	Remarks (fitness): _____ _____ _____ Remarks (personal): _____ _____ _____
Resting Pulse Rate / **Weight At Rising**			

Friday	E X E R C I S E	Activity _____ _____ Time _____ Distance _____ Pace _____ Effort: ☐ Easy ☐ Moderate ☐ Hard ☐ Extreme	Remarks (fitness): _____ _____ _____ Remarks (personal): _____ _____ _____
Resting Pulse Rate / **Weight At Rising**			

Saturday	E X E R C I S E	Activity _____ _____ Time _____ Distance _____ Pace _____ Effort: ☐ Easy ☐ Moderate ☐ Hard ☐ Extreme	Remarks (fitness): _____ _____ _____ Remarks (personal): _____ _____ _____
Resting Pulse Rate / **Weight At Rising**			

Sunday	E X E R C I S E	Activity _____ _____ Time _____ Distance _____ Pace _____ Effort: ☐ Easy ☐ Moderate ☐ Hard ☐ Extreme	Remarks (fitness): _____ _____ _____ Remarks (personal): _____ _____ _____
Resting Pulse Rate / **Weight At Rising**			

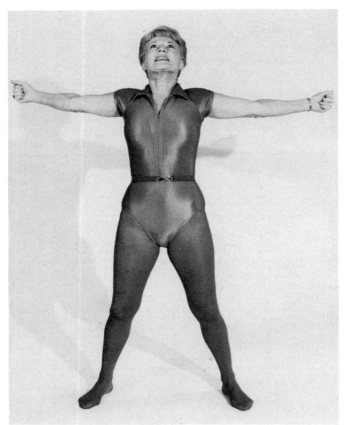

If being unfit is a long, dark corridor, reach for the brightest star.

Goals for this week:
1. _____
2. _____

Goals for this month:
1. _____
2. _____

Be an Inventor

Don't be afraid to "invent" your own exercises. Many of the best exercises I do are variations of basic exercises. In this picture, for instance, I am doing Arm Circles. But once I got going, I found it was quite a bit of fun to do variations. You can see some of the variations. They're terrific!

Energy Salad
(Wheat Bulgur Salad)

1 cup bulgur, fine grind (can be purchased by the pound at Middle-Eastern stores)
1 bunch parsley, chopped fine
1 tomato, medium, chopped fine
2-3 green onions, chopped fine
Season to taste: salt, 1 or 2 mint leaves, lemon juice, safflower oil

Soak bulgur in warm water for approximately ½ hour. Squeeze dry. Add chopped parsley and tomato. Season. Serve on lettuce leaf or stuff into tomato.

This week covers _____ , _____ , _____ , to _____ , _____ , _____ .
month   day   year   month   day   year

Monday	E X E R C I S E	Activity _____ _____ Time _____ Distance _____ Pace _____ Effort: ☐ Easy ☐ Moderate ☐ Hard ☐ Extreme	Remarks (fitness): _____ _____ _____ Remarks (personal): _____ _____ _____
Resting Pulse Rate / **Weight At Rising**			

Tuesday	E X E R C I S E	Activity _____ _____ Time _____ Distance _____ Pace _____ Effort: ☐ Easy ☐ Moderate ☐ Hard ☐ Extreme	Remarks (fitness): _____ _____ _____ Remarks (personal): _____ _____ _____
Resting Pulse Rate / **Weight At Rising**			

Wednesday	E X E R C I S E	Activity _____ _____ Time _____ Distance _____ Pace _____ Effort: ☐ Easy ☐ Moderate ☐ Hard ☐ Extreme	Remarks (fitness): _____ _____ _____ Remarks (personal): _____ _____ _____
Resting Pulse Rate / **Weight At Rising**			

Thursday	E X E R C I S E	Activity _____ _____ Time _____ Distance _____ Pace _____ Effort: ☐ Easy ☐ Moderate ☐ Hard ☐ Extreme	Remarks (fitness): _____ _____ _____ Remarks (personal): _____ _____ _____
Resting Pulse Rate / **Weight At Rising**			

Friday	E X E R C I S E	Activity _____ _____ Time _____ Distance _____ Pace _____ Effort: ☐ Easy ☐ Moderate ☐ Hard ☐ Extreme	Remarks (fitness): _____ _____ _____ Remarks (personal): _____ _____ _____
Resting Pulse Rate / **Weight At Rising**			

Saturday	E X E R C I S E	Activity _____ _____ Time _____ Distance _____ Pace _____ Effort: ☐ Easy ☐ Moderate ☐ Hard ☐ Extreme	Remarks (fitness): _____ _____ _____ Remarks (personal): _____ _____ _____
Resting Pulse Rate / **Weight At Rising**			

Sunday	E X E R C I S E	Activity _____ _____ Time _____ Distance _____ Pace _____ Effort: ☐ Easy ☐ Moderate ☐ Hard ☐ Extreme	Remarks (fitness): _____ _____ _____ Remarks (personal): _____ _____ _____
Resting Pulse Rate / **Weight At Rising**			

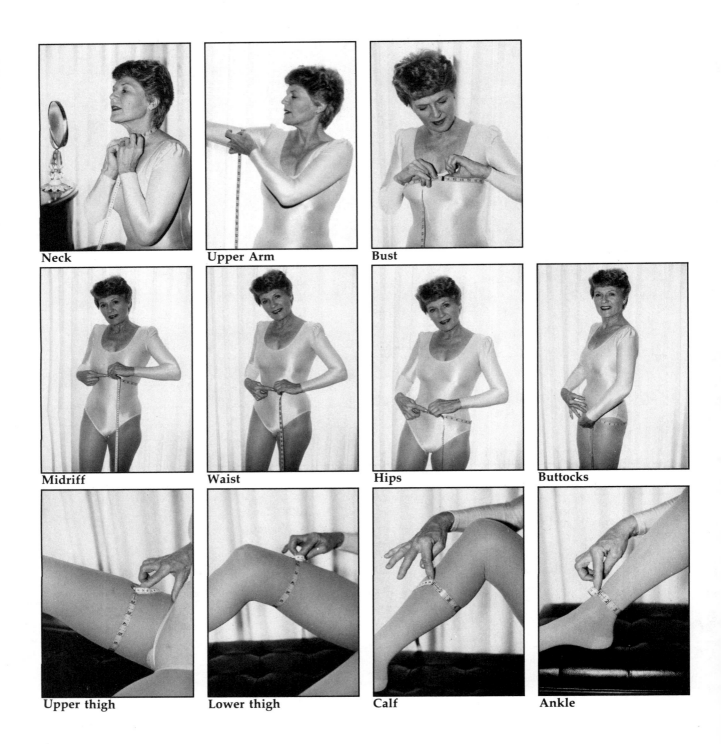

Neck

Upper Arm

Bust

Midriff

Waist

Hips

Buttocks

Upper thigh

Lower thigh

Calf

Ankle

Neck

Upper Arm

Bust

Midriff

Waist

Hips

Buttocks

Upper thigh

Lower thigh

Calf

Ankle

You have yet to meet the person of full potential that you can be.

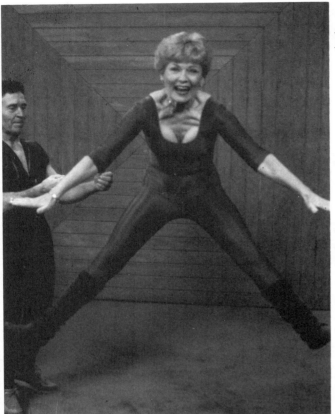

Let Yourself Fly
This one might look to some of you as though Jack had just pointed out that there was a mouse in front of the cameraman, but he didn't. We were exhibiting, on our TV show, some of the fun you can have doing jumps and spreads once you've gotten yourself into shape. One of the things I like about getting fit is that it allows you to act a lot less than your chronological age.

Goals for this week:
1. _____
2. _____

Goals for this month:
1. _____
2. _____

Baked Custard

4 eggs, slightly beaten
¾-1½ cups honey (depending on taste)
2½ cups non-fat milk
½ tsp. salt
½ tsp. vanilla
nutmeg (optional: before baking, you may sprinkle on top)

Mix ingredients and oven poach at 350 degrees until knife comes out clean from center of custard. (Note: To oven poach, set individual cups or large baking dish in a baking pan with a bit of water.)

This week covers _____ , _____ , _____ , to _____ , _____ , _____ .
month   day   year   month   day   year

Monday

Resting Pulse Rate	Weight At Rising

EXERCISE

Activity _____

_____

Time _____

Distance _____

Pace _____

Effort: ☐ Easy ☐ Moderate ☐ Hard ☐ Extreme

Remarks (fitness): _____

_____

_____

Remarks (personal): _____

_____

_____

Tuesday

Resting Pulse Rate	Weight At Rising

EXERCISE

Activity _____

_____

Time _____

Distance _____

Pace _____

Effort: ☐ Easy ☐ Moderate ☐ Hard ☐ Extreme

Remarks (fitness): _____

_____

_____

Remarks (personal): _____

_____

_____

Wednesday

Resting Pulse Rate	Weight At Rising

EXERCISE

Activity _____

_____

Time _____

Distance _____

Pace _____

Effort: ☐ Easy ☐ Moderate ☐ Hard ☐ Extreme

Remarks (fitness): _____

_____

_____

Remarks (personal): _____

_____

_____

Thursday

Resting Pulse Rate	Weight At Rising

EXERCISE

Activity _____

_____

Time _____

Distance _____

Pace _____

Effort: ☐ Easy ☐ Moderate ☐ Hard ☐ Extreme

Remarks (fitness): _____

_____

_____

Remarks (personal): _____

_____

_____

Friday

Resting Pulse Rate	Weight At Rising

EXERCISE

Activity _____

_____

Time _____

Distance _____

Pace _____

Effort: ☐ Easy ☐ Moderate ☐ Hard ☐ Extreme

Remarks (fitness): _____

_____

_____

Remarks (personal): _____

_____

_____

Saturday

Resting Pulse Rate	Weight At Rising

EXERCISE

Activity _____

_____

Time _____

Distance _____

Pace _____

Effort: ☐ Easy ☐ Moderate ☐ Hard ☐ Extreme

Remarks (fitness): _____

_____

_____

Remarks (personal): _____

_____

_____

Sunday

Resting Pulse Rate	Weight At Rising

EXERCISE

Activity _____

_____

Time _____

Distance _____

Pace _____

Effort: ☐ Easy ☐ Moderate ☐ Hard ☐ Extreme

Remarks (fitness): _____

_____

_____

Remarks (personal): _____

_____

_____

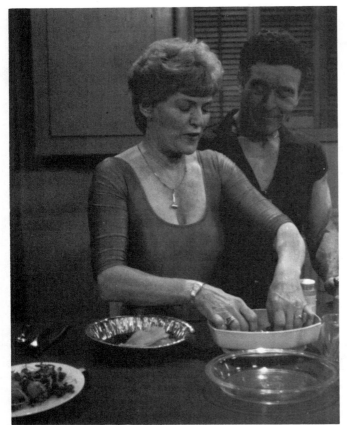

A one-mile run before you go to work puts you a mile ahead of everyone else all day.

Goals for this week:

1. _____

2. _____

Goals for this month:

1. _____

2. _____

Good Food

Don't overlook the importance of good nutrition. As I've said at several other places in this book, you don't have to get into exotic and difficult-to-follow diets. Merely concentrate on cutting down your intake of foods that you know are bad for you. Learn to love foods in their natural state.

Broiled Filet of Sole

1 large filet of sole (sliced in half, down the middle) or small pieces of Dover sole
¼ cup soy sauce
⅛ cup safflower oil
garlic powder
fresh parsley
season to taste

Take fish filet and marinate 30 seconds to one minute in sauce and then roll up around parsley springs. Use toothpicks to keep together. Parsley should extend from edges as colorful garnish. Broil approximately 5–10 minutes—do not overbroil. *Sauce to marinate:* mix soy sauce, oil, and seasoning together and set fish in flat dish to soak in flavor.

This week covers _____ , _____ , _____ , to _____ , _____ , _____ .
month   day   year   month   day   year

Monday

Resting Pulse Rate	Weight At Rising

E X E R C I S E

Activity _____
_____
Time _____
Distance _____
Pace _____
Effort: ☐ Easy   ☐ Moderate
       ☐ Hard   ☐ Extreme

Remarks (fitness): _____
_____
Remarks (personal): _____
_____

Tuesday

Resting Pulse Rate	Weight At Rising

E X E R C I S E

Activity _____
_____
Time _____
Distance _____
Pace _____
Effort: ☐ Easy   ☐ Moderate
       ☐ Hard   ☐ Extreme

Remarks (fitness): _____
_____
Remarks (personal): _____
_____

Wednesday

Resting Pulse Rate	Weight At Rising

E X E R C I S E

Activity _____
_____
Time _____
Distance _____
Pace _____
Effort: ☐ Easy   ☐ Moderate
       ☐ Hard   ☐ Extreme

Remarks (fitness): _____
_____
Remarks (personal): _____
_____

Thursday

Resting Pulse Rate	Weight At Rising

E X E R C I S E

Activity _____
_____
Time _____
Distance _____
Pace _____
Effort: ☐ Easy   ☐ Moderate
       ☐ Hard   ☐ Extreme

Remarks (fitness): _____
_____
Remarks (personal): _____
_____

Friday

Resting Pulse Rate	Weight At Rising

E X E R C I S E

Activity _____
_____
Time _____
Distance _____
Pace _____
Effort: ☐ Easy   ☐ Moderate
       ☐ Hard   ☐ Extreme

Remarks (fitness): _____
_____
Remarks (personal): _____
_____

Saturday

Resting Pulse Rate	Weight At Rising

E X E R C I S E

Activity _____
_____
Time _____
Distance _____
Pace _____
Effort: ☐ Easy   ☐ Moderate
       ☐ Hard   ☐ Extreme

Remarks (fitness): _____
_____
Remarks (personal): _____
_____

Sunday

Resting Pulse Rate	Weight At Rising

E X E R C I S E

Activity _____
_____
Time _____
Distance _____
Pace _____
Effort: ☐ Easy   ☐ Moderate
       ☐ Hard   ☐ Extreme

Remarks (fitness): _____
_____
Remarks (personal): _____
_____

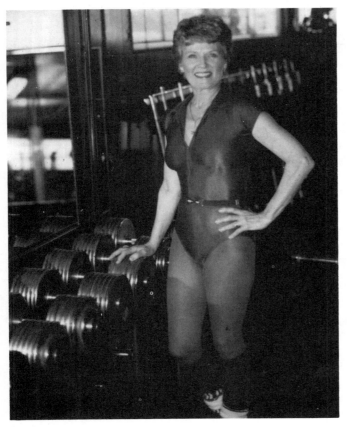

Using Weights
Jack and I have always believed in the opportunity to reshape your body by the careful use of weights. We have a complete set in our home that we use every morning. They provide a real route to making a significant inroad to your goals. Don't overlook them as a means to a new you.

Goals for this week:
1. _____
2. _____
Goals for this month:
1. _____
2. _____

Get into the swim of fitness—even if you start by dog-paddling.

Cheese-topped Zucchini Halves

3 medium (or 5 small) zucchini squash
1 medium onion (thinly sliced)
1 tbsp. salad oil
½ to 1 tsp. crushed oregano
1 cup seasoned tomato sauce
1 6- or 8-oz. package sliced Mozzarella cheese (or mild cheddar)
grated Parmesan cheese

Cut (same size) zucchini in half lengthwise, and place them in an oiled baking dish approximately 8×12, cut side up. Top with grated cheddar cheese, onion, oregano and tomato sauce. Bake until tender or chewy in 350 degree oven. You can also double the recipe and put a second layer on top of the first and bake until tender. Sprinkle with Parmesan cheese. *Variation:* Ground beef or ground turkey can be added.

This week covers _____ , _____ , _____ , to _____ , _____ , _____ .
month   day   year   month   day   year

Monday	E X E R C I S E	Activity _____ _____ Time _____ Distance _____ Pace _____ Effort: ☐ Easy ☐ Moderate ☐ Hard ☐ Extreme	Remarks (fitness): _____ _____ _____ Remarks (personal): _____ _____ _____
Resting Pulse Rate / **Weight At Rising**			

Tuesday	E X E R C I S E	Activity _____ _____ Time _____ Distance _____ Pace _____ Effort: ☐ Easy ☐ Moderate ☐ Hard ☐ Extreme	Remarks (fitness): _____ _____ _____ Remarks (personal): _____ _____ _____
Resting Pulse Rate / **Weight At Rising**			

Wednesday	E X E R C I S E	Activity _____ _____ Time _____ Distance _____ Pace _____ Effort: ☐ Easy ☐ Moderate ☐ Hard ☐ Extreme	Remarks (fitness): _____ _____ _____ Remarks (personal): _____ _____ _____
Resting Pulse Rate / **Weight At Rising**			

Thursday	E X E R C I S E	Activity _____ _____ Time _____ Distance _____ Pace _____ Effort: ☐ Easy ☐ Moderate ☐ Hard ☐ Extreme	Remarks (fitness): _____ _____ _____ Remarks (personal): _____ _____ _____
Resting Pulse Rate / **Weight At Rising**			

Friday	E X E R C I S E	Activity _____ _____ Time _____ Distance _____ Pace _____ Effort: ☐ Easy ☐ Moderate ☐ Hard ☐ Extreme	Remarks (fitness): _____ _____ _____ Remarks (personal): _____ _____ _____
Resting Pulse Rate / **Weight At Rising**			

Saturday	E X E R C I S E	Activity _____ _____ Time _____ Distance _____ Pace _____ Effort: ☐ Easy ☐ Moderate ☐ Hard ☐ Extreme	Remarks (fitness): _____ _____ _____ Remarks (personal): _____ _____ _____
Resting Pulse Rate / **Weight At Rising**			

Sunday	E X E R C I S E	Activity _____ _____ Time _____ Distance _____ Pace _____ Effort: ☐ Easy ☐ Moderate ☐ Hard ☐ Extreme	Remarks (fitness): _____ _____ _____ Remarks (personal): _____ _____ _____
Resting Pulse Rate / **Weight At Rising**			

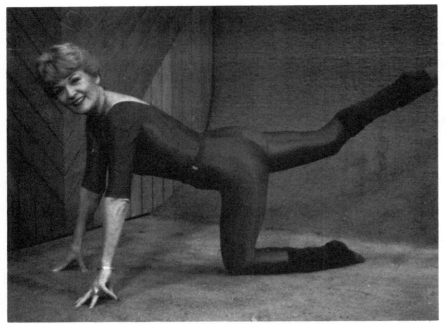

Stay Happy

This is a review. We've gone over this exercise before. But I'm putting it in, not as an exercise, but as my graphic way of saying to you, from the heart: "Get a kick out of life by getting serious about fitness for the rest of your life. Kick the unfitness habit, and make yourself as strong as a mule. Stay fit, stay active, stay happy."

Goals for this week:

1. _____
2. _____

Goals for this month:

1. _____
2. _____

The only down people are those who haven't looked up lately.

Potatoes LaLanne

1 medium potato
safflower oil
seasoning to taste

Wash potato with skin. Scrub carefully as though for baking. Then dry. Slice potatoes crosswise in approximately 1/8-inch thickness, leaving skin on. Dip each slice in mixture of safflower oil and season, according to taste, with vegetable seasoning, garlic and/or onion powder. Place each slice separately on a large sheet of foil (laid on a cookie sheet), crimping the edges. Place in the broiler, which has been pre-heated for five minutes. Broil 3-5 minutes until crispy brown. Flip the slices and brown the other side. Serve with meal or as a substitute for potato chips.

This week covers _____ , _____ , _____ , to _____ , _____ , _____ .
month   day   year   month   day   year

Monday	E X E R C I S E	Activity _____ _____ Time _____ Distance _____ Pace _____ Effort: ☐ Easy ☐ Moderate ☐ Hard ☐ Extreme	Remarks (fitness): _____ _____ _____ Remarks (personal): _____ _____ _____
Resting Pulse Rate / **Weight At Rising**			

Tuesday	E X E R C I S E	Activity _____ _____ Time _____ Distance _____ Pace _____ Effort: ☐ Easy ☐ Moderate ☐ Hard ☐ Extreme	Remarks (fitness): _____ _____ _____ Remarks (personal): _____ _____ _____
Resting Pulse Rate / **Weight At Rising**			

Wednesday	E X E R C I S E	Activity _____ _____ Time _____ Distance _____ Pace _____ Effort: ☐ Easy ☐ Moderate ☐ Hard ☐ Extreme	Remarks (fitness): _____ _____ _____ Remarks (personal): _____ _____ _____
Resting Pulse Rate / **Weight At Rising**			

Thursday	E X E R C I S E	Activity _____ _____ Time _____ Distance _____ Pace _____ Effort: ☐ Easy ☐ Moderate ☐ Hard ☐ Extreme	Remarks (fitness): _____ _____ _____ Remarks (personal): _____ _____ _____
Resting Pulse Rate / **Weight At Rising**			

Friday	E X E R C I S E	Activity _____ _____ Time _____ Distance _____ Pace _____ Effort: ☐ Easy ☐ Moderate ☐ Hard ☐ Extreme	Remarks (fitness): _____ _____ _____ Remarks (personal): _____ _____ _____
Resting Pulse Rate / **Weight At Rising**			

Saturday	E X E R C I S E	Activity _____ _____ Time _____ Distance _____ Pace _____ Effort: ☐ Easy ☐ Moderate ☐ Hard ☐ Extreme	Remarks (fitness): _____ _____ _____ Remarks (personal): _____ _____ _____
Resting Pulse Rate / **Weight At Rising**			

Sunday	E X E R C I S E	Activity _____ _____ Time _____ Distance _____ Pace _____ Effort: ☐ Easy ☐ Moderate ☐ Hard ☐ Extreme	Remarks (fitness): _____ _____ _____ Remarks (personal): _____ _____ _____
Resting Pulse Rate / **Weight At Rising**			

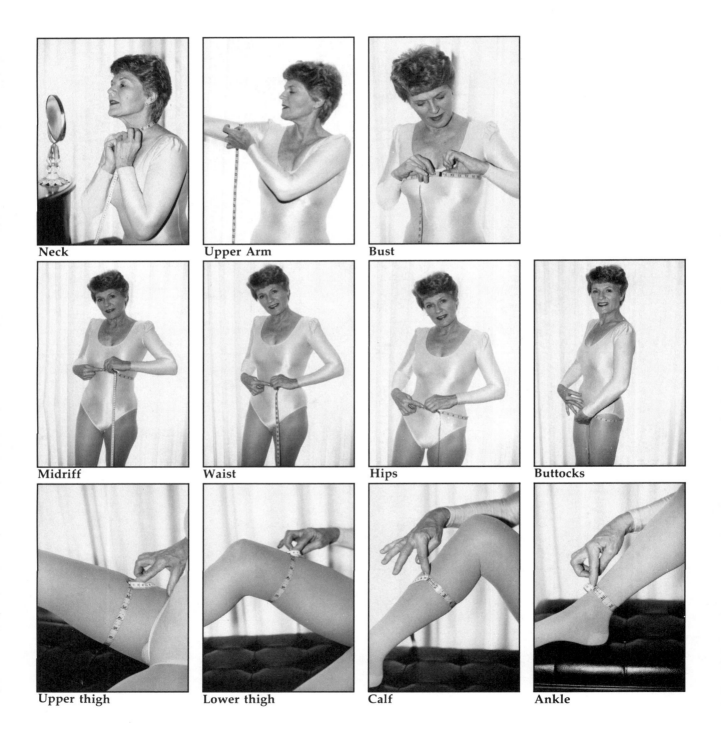

Neck

Upper Arm

Bust

Midriff

Waist

Hips

Buttocks

Upper thigh

Lower thigh

Calf

Ankle

Neck

Upper Arm

Bust

Midriff

Waist

Hips

Buttocks

Upper thigh

Lower thigh

Calf

Ankle

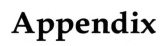

Appendix

Spring meal plan

No fitness program can sustain itself well over an entire year without periodic re-evaluation and re-setting of your goals. It should also have regularly scheduled points where progress is measured, and where the exerciser can celebrate a victory along the way. With this *Diary*, it does not matter when you begin your program—you can jump right in on any week of the year. Neither does it matter when you come upon your seasonal celebration. If it's summer when you complete your first three months' worth of exercising, just go to the summer meal plan and either invite a few friends over to help you celebrate your victory, or quietly celebrate it by yourself, using it as an opportunity to review how you've done over the last three months in keeping to your goals, and coming up with new goals for the upcoming three months.

For your Spring Meal Plan, these are the suggested foods for your very special day. Of course, you are free to substitute in whatever you wish. These are only suggestions:

Breakfast: 4 oz. Apple Juice
Banana Toast
Lunch: Blender Soup
Dinner: Glazed Chicken with Mustard Sauce
Elaine's Rice Dish
Bean Sprout Salad
Date Nut Squares

Banana Toast

½ to 1 whole banana
1 egg
1 slice whole grain bread
season to taste with mace, nutmeg, cinnamon

Put banana in blender or mash. Add egg and spices. Mix well. Dip slice of bread in mixture and brown slightly on each side in a nonstick pan or griddle. (Similar to French Toast.)

Blender Soup

1 can chicken broth or homemade chicken stock
1 carrot, chopped
½ zucchini, chopped
1 small bell pepper, chopped
1 stalk celery, chopped

Mix the above ingredients in blender. Pour in saucepan and bring to boil. (Note: You may substitute any of the vegetables mentioned for the ones you have sitting in your refrigerator waiting to be used.) Serves 2 or 3.
Variation:
1 cup water
1 can chicken broth
¾ cup each of celery, bell pepper, potato, cauliflower, carrots, cucumber, zucchini (all chopped)

Heat and serve.

Glazed Chicken with Mustard Sauce

6 chicken legs with thighs
slivered almonds

Place 6 legs with thighs in greased baking dish. Cover with mustard sauce (recipe below) and bake at 400 degrees for half an hour. Sprinkle with slivered almonds and leave in oven with temperature off for another 10 minutes. At this initial baking, you may taste periodically.

Mustard Sauce for Chicken

½ cup honey
½ cup Grey Poupon Dijon mustard
1 tsp. lemon juice
1 tsp. onion
½ tsp. curry powder

Mix ingredients in small bowl until thoroughly mixed together.

Elaine's Rice Dish

2 cups cooked brown rice
1 cup celery
1 cup bell pepper
1 cup chopped onion
1 cup mushrooms
garlic powder to taste
vegetable seasoning to taste

Lightly saute celery, bell pepper, onions, and mushrooms. Add cooked rice. Season with garlic and your own seasonings to taste. Note: The secret to this recipe is not to overcook the vegetables. Keep them crisp!

Bean Sprout Salad

2 cups fresh bean sprouts
1 cup celery, sliced thin
1 cup radishes, sliced thin
4 scallions, sliced
Dressing:
¾ cup oil
⅛ cup vinegar
¼ cup soy sauce

Mix together oil, vinegar and soy sauce. Pour over vegetables. However, do not use entire amount, as it may be too much for this amount of vegetables; this depends on your taste.

Date and Nut Squares

2 eggs
⅓ cup honey
½ tsp. vanilla
½ cup flour
½ tsp. baking powder
1 cup walnuts, chopped
2 cups dates, finely chopped

Beat eggs until foamy. Beat in honey and vanilla. Mix in remaining ingredients. Put into an oiled and floured 8-inch square pan and bake at 375 degrees for approximately 25-30 minutes, or until top has dull crust. Cut into squares and cool. Remove from pan. Makes 12 squares.

Summer meal plan

Summer is the time for a radical increase in outdoor activity. It is the time for going to the beach, for playing baseball, for playing Frisbee, for just generally getting out of the house and doing things. Few people can resist the attraction of summer. And this is a very good thing, because all of this increase in activity generally has a healthy effect on people, because the activity causes them to use more calories (and consequently, to lose a little weight) and build muscle tone. The summer is a terrific time to schedule one of your four seasonal celebrations, and let me suggest that you do it at some significant point in the summer. For instance, how about the first day of summer? Or how about the weekend before the big Fourth of July weekend? (That way you can celebrate your accomplishments and look forward to the next three-month period without it being overwhelmed by the big holiday, and you can go into the July Fourth holiday with your new goals in place.) Or perhaps you can do it at the mid-point of July, roughly halfway through the traditional Memorial Day to Labor Day summer.

For your Summer Meal Plan, these are the suggested foods. Substitute as you feel necessary, but keep it light and cheery:

Breakfast: LaLanne's Frothy
Elaine's Wheat Germ Muffins
Lunch: Jon's Quick Lunch
Dinner: Broiled Filet of Sole
Wheat Pilaf
Fruit Salad

LaLanne's Frothy

4-5 oz. apple juice, unfiltered
4-5 oz. milk, raw or non-fat
3-4 tbsp. protein powder
2 tbsp. raw wheat germ
1 tbsp. natural bran
1 tbsp. brewer's yeast
½ small banana, very ripe
honey or fructose for sweetening if desired
ice, small amount, if desired

Put all ingredients into blender, whip until frothy and all items have mixed thoroughly.

Elaine's Wheat Germ Muffins

¼ cup bran
1 cup raw wheat germ
⅔ cup milk
1 egg
¾ cup safflower oil
1 cup whole wheat flour (sifted)
2½ tsp. baking powder
¼ cup honey
½ cup raisins

Sift whole wheat flour and baking powder together and then add other ingredients. Mix together. Bake in moderate oven (400 degrees) about 25 minutes. *Variation:* Add nuts, berries, or dried fruits.

Jon LaLanne's Quick Lunch

lettuce
drained sardines or water pack tuna
tomato slices
2 heaping tbsp. cottage cheese
whole wheat crackers

On a bed of lettuce, arrange sardines or tuna with tomato slices. Top with cottage cheese, and serve with whole wheat crackers.

Broiled Filet of Sole

1 large filet of sole (sliced in half, down the middle) or small pieces of Dover sole
¼ cup soy sauce
⅛ cup safflower oil
garlic powder
fresh parsley
season to taste

Take fish filet and marinate 30 seconds to one minute in sauce and then roll up around parsley sprigs. Use toothpicks to keep together. Parsley should extend from edges as colorful garnish. Broil approximately 5–10 minutes—do not overbroil. *Sauce to marinate:* Mix soy sauce, oil, and seasoning together and set fish in flat dish to soak in flavor.

Wheat Pilaf

safflower oil
handful vermicelli noodles
1½ cups coarse wheat (bulgar)
14½-oz. can chicken broth or your chicken stock
1 cup water
2 cubes chicken or beef bouillon

In safflower oil, brown vermicelli noodles, stirring constantly so as not to burn. Keep stirring, then add wheat to vermicelli. Pour in broth, water and bouillon cubes and bring to a quick boil. Lower heat and simmer with cover until liquid is gone. Let set before serving.

Fruit Salad

3 lettuce leaves, torn
1 medium apple, with peel, diced
6 grapes (red, green or black)
raisins, sunflower seeds, nuts (optional)
dressing: 1 cup yogurt, thinned with 2 tbsp. fruit juice (concentrate)

Place lettuce in plate, arrange apple and grapes. Top with dressing and sprinkle with raisins, sunflower seeds, nuts, etc.

Autumn meal plan

In many parts of the country, autumn is the most beautiful time of the year—bar none. It is also a time of the year when many active people get their last flings in with outdoor activities before the bad weather of winter sets in. It is a time for those last picnics, cycle trips, running those fall marathons, taking hikes. And it is also a time for getting ready for the next season by signing up for aerobic dance classes, oiling the indoor exercise equipment, and planning a vigorous exercise program to augment what you've been doing over the summer. So take a day during the fall, plan it well in advance, and use it as the day when you celebrate a successful summer season coming to a close, and your embarking on a joyful and active fall season. Perhaps invite a few friends by and compare notes about all of the marvelous things you did over the summer, and how it seemed to literally fly by. And perhaps discuss what your plans are for a fabulous fall and the things that you can serve on that very special day of looking back at what you've accomplished and looking ahead at what you plan to do are these:

Breakfast: 1/2 Cantaloupe
Scrambled Eggs and Salsa
Lunch: 4 oz. Consomme
Carrot Raisin Pineapple Salad
Dinner: Wheat Soya Spaghetti with Clams
Dilled Peppers and Cukes
Yogurt/Banana Freeze

Scrambled Eggs and Salsa

1 zucchini, chopped
2-3 mushrooms, chopped (optional)
1 green onion, tops chopped
1 tomato, chopped
1 heart of celery stalks, chopped
4 eggs

Sauté the vegetables in 1 tbsp. oil; add tomato last. Scramble 4 eggs in separate frying pan. Serve eggs in individual platters, garnish with parsley and top with above salsa.

Carrot Raisin Pineapple Salad

2 cups grated carrots
½ cup raisins or currants
½ cup pineapple chunks
¼ cup honey
¼ cup oil
¼ cup lemon juice
¼ cup chopped walnuts

Toss all together. Place on lettuce leaves. Grated apple can also be added.

Wheat-Soya Spaghetti

2 cups cooked wheat-soya spaghetti
1 6½-oz. portion of chopped clams
and/or shrimp or scallops
½ cup chopped tomatoes (preferably
fresh)

In a frying pan, mix above together until desired warmth. Season to taste. *Variation:* Add mushrooms and grated carrots.

Dilled Peppers and Cukes

red pepper rings
scored sliced cucumbers

Arrange pepper rings and cucumbers on bed of watercress. Top with Dill Dressing.

Dill Dressing:

1 tbsp. mayonnaise
1 tbsp. yogurt (plain)
dill weed to taste

Mix all ingredients and serve.

Yogurt-Banana Freeze

2 cups very ripe bananas
1½ cups plain yogurt

Put in blender and mix well. Pour into ice cube trays and freeze. Before serving, put pieces through blender again. (This will make it appear like soft ice cream or frozen yogurt.) *Variations:* Add pineapple (fresh or canned) to mixture in blender after freezing. You may use any fruit desired; however, pineapple will give a sweeter flavor. You may also add apple, orange or pineapple juices. Experiment with this one; be creative.

Winter meal plan

In the cycle of the human body, there seems to come a time when it must rest. In a seasonal sort of way, nature takes care of that much-needed rest by making it difficult to be overly active in the winter. All of the muscles and joints that work so hard to help you maintain your fitness during the rest of the year get a needed rest so they can rebuild themselves. Now don't take me wrong on this count. I'm not saying that you should be encouraged to vegetate all winter. I'm merely saying that in nature, winter indicates a time to back off a bit, allow yourself to regroup, and it provides a perfect time to retire indoors and do indoor exercises, play racquetball and other such pursuits. I'm also very fond of the Thanksgiving and Christmas Holidays, and I don't see anything wrong with indulging a bit in those festive seasons, which is one way you're bound to slow down your usual progress toward staying fit. During this period, pick fitness activities that will allow you to enjoy your home a little more. I enjoy doing a regular series of workouts at home during the winter, and then I love to spend time in the kitchen. Pick one weekend during the winter when you can prepare your day of looking back at the fall and looking ahead to your goals this winter, and put together a nice day's worth of meals. Here are some suggestions:

Breakfast: 1/2 Grapefruit
High Protein Pancakes
Lunch: Bulgar Salad
Dinner: Lamb Stew
White Radish and Jicama Salad
Poached Pears/Apples

High-Protein Pancakes

4 eggs
1 cup cottage cheese
2 tbsp. safflower oil
¼ cup oatmeal (or ¼ cup wheat germ & ¼ cup oatmeal)
¼ tsp. salt

Place all ingredients in a blender and mix thoroughly. Drop by tablespoon onto hot greased frying pan or griddle. Serves 3-4. *Variation:* ½ cup whole wheat flour may also be used instead of oatmeal.

Energy Salad (Wheat Bulgur Salad)

1 cup bulgur, fine grind (can be purchased by the pound at Middle-Eastern stores)
1 bunch parsley, chopped fine
1 tomato, medium, chopped fine
2-3 green onions, chopped fine
Season to taste: salt, 1 or 2 mint leaves, lemon juice, safflower oil

Soak bulgur in warm water for approximately ½ hour. Squeeze dry. Add chopped parsley and tomato. Season. Serve on lettuce leaf or stuff in tomato.

Lamb Stew

1 lb. lamb stew meat (neck or
  shoulder cut)
½ cup mushrooms
1 cup turnips
1 cup zucchini
1 cup potatoes, sliced
1 cup carrots
1 cup celery
1 medium onion
2 cups fresh tomatoes (or 1 can
  stewed tomatoes)

Brown lamb and onion in a large skillet, season with garlic powder, crumpled bay leaf and favorite seasonings. Pour over tomatoes, simmer until tender. (You may have to add a little water or beef broth as you stew the lamb, depending upon how much moisture you lose.) When lamb is tender, add vegetables and simmer until they are done but still crispy. *Variation:* Cooked brown rice may be used instead of potatoes. *Quick Stew:* If your lamb is tender you may like to just brown the lamb until it is pink inside. Sauté your vegetables in separate skillet until you can barely put a fork in them. Add tomatoes, heat through and then add your lamb last. Season the same as above.

White Radish and Jicama Salad

1 cup grated white radish
¼ cup grated carrot
¼ cup grated jicama
1 cucumber

Arrange grated vegetables on lettuce leaves in layers. Slice cucumber with peel and arrange around plate. Top with dressing. For fancy slices, score cucumber.

Poached Pears or Apples

3 firm, ripe pears (use apples if
  pears aren't in season)
¾ cup honey
¾ cup water
1 tsp. lemon juice
1 tsp. vanilla extract

Core pears or apples and cut in half, leaving skins on. Combine honey, water, lemon juice and vanilla in saucepan, and bring to a boil. Add fruit, reduce heat and cook for approximately 20 minutes. Chill and serve with kiwi slices.

Aerobic sports guide

The majority of the fitness revolution that has been sweeping America is centered on aerobic fitness activities.

In order for the cells of the body (i.e., muscle cells, pancreas cells, etc.) to perform their respective functions, energy is required. This needed energy is derived from the metabolism (breakdown) of the foodstuffs (primarily carbohydrates) that we eat. This energy formation occurs in two ways—through anaerobic and aerobic metabolism.

The energy yielded as a result of anaerobic processes results without utilizing oxygen in metabolizing our food. Without the utilization of oxygen, the body turns to pulling glycogen (energy) directly from the liver and muscles where it is stored. This energy is delivered to muscles much more rapidly than during aerobic processes. However, the human body can only function in this fashion for a short period of time, for the liver and muscle glycogen stores become rapidly depleted. Consequently, any energy used in strenuous bursts of activity lasting more than a few seconds but less than two minutes is anaerobic in nature.

On the other hand, aerobic energy is that which can be derived from foods by using oxygen. Although provided more slowly than anaerobic energy, aerobic energy is almost inexhaustible so muscles can be trained to perform a long, long time.

For example, if you sprint to catch a bus (and you become out of breath), that is anaerobic exercise. If, on the other hand, you see from some blocks away that you'll never catch the bus if you don't pick up the pace, but then you merely dog-trot along for three minutes (your breath never coming in desperate gasps), that's aerobic.

Hopefully, this illustrates how a workout which is generally considered to be anaerobic in nature (short, intermittent bursts of varying repetitious activity) can become quite an aerobic session when performed slower but non-stop. The most important muscle in the body, the heart, receives quite a workout and becomes stronger and more efficient (accomplishes an equal or greater amount of work with less effort) in the process. It is this increased efficiency which offers protection against heart attacks for, in a stressful situation, the strong heart is better able to meet the body's needs than is a weak one.

There are also other benefits. Regular aerobic exercise is an excellent way of relieving stress that builds up in modern man's daily life. It tones the muscles. It can be used in conjunction with a careful food regimen to lose weight. And, many types of aerobic activities can be just plain fun.

Back in 1968, my friend Dr. Ken Cooper made America aware of the aerobic concept by publishing a book called, simply *Aerobics*. The book outlined a fitness program that used aerobic sports and activities. It promoted constant movement at a level that is comfortable.

We're not going to go into a long study of aerobic activities here. If you want more information on aerobic activities, you can find plenty of good information in Dr. Cooper's excellent books. What we are going to do is to merely look briefly at some of the more popular aerobic exercises, and make some comments on them. And then you're on your own.

Walking. By far, the easiest of all aerobic exercises to perform. The walking program can begin as a very modest program and, as you become more and more fit, can become much more ambitious. When you walk, continue walking the entire time; don't stop and chat with people; walk briskly and with authority. Start by setting time goals, and not goals of distance. Also remember that a day when you walk for a long time should be followed by a day where you walk a short time, so that your body can recover. Walking can be done at virtually any time, at any place. Minimum stress is placed on the bones and joints. Walking can be incorporated easily into daily life, and it can be done alone.

Jogging/Running. One of the most popular aerobic fitness activities in this country, and it's rapidly catching on in England, Europe, Australia, New Zealand, Japan, and many other countries. Jogging is slow running, or the act of running along slowly, with almost as much energy spent bouncing up and down as is used to move forward. Running is smoother, more concentrated, and is done at a relatively faster pace. You can jog at almost any time, and at almost any place. You don't need a partner and you don't have to reserve a court. It very quickly builds up aerobic fitness. Be sure, however, to invest in a good pair of running shoes if you are going to take up this activity. Your feet and legs will thank you.

Cycling. Cycling helps build leg muscles and can be worked into a person's commute to work, or can be done as a weekend fun activity. For benefits, however, it must be done regularly (four days a week) and the rider must be exerting him- or herself during the ride. Cycling can be easily incorporated into a person's life as a means of transportation. It is a fuel-efficient and ecologically acceptable way of taking short trips.

Swimming. This is Jack's favorite activity. There is a great difference between a ''bather'' and a ''swimmer,'' however. A ''bather'' merely goes into the water, splashes around and gets wet, and that's about it. A ''swimmer'' is one who actively *swims* when in the water. As in, ''Hey, I'll race you out to that diving platform and back.'' Swimming is one of the gentlest of all the aerobic sports. There is no bashing or jolting of the joints or feet as there is in some of the other aerobic sports. You glide along and you are buoyed by the water, taking most of the pressure off your body. Swimming that is done regularly and with vigor builds fair leg strength and plenty of upper-body strength, benefitting almost every muscle in your body.

Aerobic Dancing. One of the most popular forms of exercise to come along in a long time. Primarily for women at first, but now being enjoyed by both sexes. This is a good, fun way to get aerobic exercise into your day, while also providing an opportunity to socialize with people interested in doing the same things for their bodies that you're doing for yours.

Weight Training. At first glance, you'd think that weight training doesn't fit the aerobic exercise mold. But, Jack LaLanne was the first person to begin doing aerobic weight training —way back in 1936. He encouraged his students to keep the lifting going, moving quickly and smoothly from one set of lifts to the next with a bare minimum of rest between sets. This turned weight training into an aerobic exercise. Today it is all the rage. I know for myself that I did not get the results I desired until Jack put me on a progressive, scientific program of weight training; and then I saw results—in just a few weeks. With weight training, you can isolate virtually any one of your 640 muscles and work on it specifically. You can, therefore, concentrate on your deficiencies, adjusting weights to your current strength. As you build yourself up, you can add weights. Weight training firms, tightens, tones, and increases strength. Since strength is energy, it naturally builds your energy reserves. The fact that most records in sports competition, on a world level, have been broken within the past few years is due to the fact that most athletes are incorporating a good weight training program into their overall training. Whether it's marathon runners or swimmers, they're learning that a well-rounded program makes them more efficient. Take for instance two clones: if Clone A is stronger than Clone B, Clone A will be the better performer. It is important to change your program every several weeks, due to the fact that when a muscle gets used to an exercise, it doesn't respond as well and tends to quit improving. I see weight training as an aerobic sport that can do wonders for you.

Calories burned chart

Everyone who diets is super-conscious of the word "calories."

Calories play their role in the human body, and they are very, very important to living a healthful life. Food is fuel and the body needs fuel to live and to move. Calories are merely a measurement of that process. There are about 3500 calories in one pound of fat. In other words, if you want to lose one pound of fat, you must burn 3500 calories *more* than you normally burn. Or you can ingest 3500 calories *less* than you normally do. It's quite simple: If you are taking in more calories than you are burning up, you're not going to lose weight. In fact, you'll gain weight. So regardless of what anyone says, calories *do* count. Remember: You'll never lose weight if you exceed the feed limit.

Keep in mind that calories are being burned by the living human body 24 hours a day. Even when we sleep. (One advantage of regular aerobic exercise is that the more regular the exerciser's activity, the easier calories are burned because the body adjusts to your exercise and your body burns calories at a more rapid rate even when you're sleeping than in a sedentary person.) Keep in mind also that a larger person burns more calories doing the same activity than a smaller person.

The chart that follows is a very interesting look at calories burned. We start with activities that burn very few calories and we progress to activities that burn more and more. In the middle column are your basic everyday activities and on the far right are recreational activities that burn a like number of calories. This chart is based on a person weighing about 150 pounds and it is built upon the chart carried in the book *Physical Activity and Cardiovascular Health,* by Fox, Naughton and Gorman.

Calories Per Minute	Daily Life	Recreational
2-2½	Desk work Auto driving (calmly) Typing, electric Electrical calculating machine operation	Walking (strolling 1 mile/hr.) Flying, motorcycling (calmly) Playing cards (calmly) Sewing, knitting
2½-4	Auto repair Radio, TV repair Janitorial work Typing, manual Bartending	Level walking (2 miles/hr.) Level bicycling (5 miles/hr.) Riding lawn mower Billiards, bowling Skeet, shuffleboard Woodworking (light) Powerboat driving (calmly) Golf (with power card) Canoeing (2½ miles/hr.) Horseback riding (walk) Playing piano and many musical instruments
4-5	Brick laying, plastering Wheelbarrow (100 lb. load) Machine assembly Trailer-truck in traffic Welding (moderate load) Cleaning windows	Walking (3 miles/hr.) Cycling (6 miles/hr.) Horseshoe pitching Volleyball (6-man noncompetitive) Golf (pulling bag cart) Archery Sailing (handling small boat) Fly fishing (standing with waders) Horseback (sitting to trot) Badminton (social doubles) Pushing light power mower Energetic musician

Calories Per Minute	Daily Life	Recreational
5-6	Painting, masonry Paperhanging Light carpentry	Walking (3½ miles/hr.) Cycling (8 miles/hr.) Table tennis Golf (carrying clubs) Dancing (foxtrot) Badminton (singles) Tennis (doubles) Raking leaves Hoeing Many calisthenics
6-7	Digging garden Shoveling light earth	Walking (4 miles/hr.) Cycling (10 miles/hr.) Canoeing (4 miles/hr.) Horseback ("posting" to trot) Stream fishing (walking in light current in waders) Ice or roller skating (9 miles/hr.)
7-8	Shoveling at 10 lifts per minute (10-pound lifts)	Walking (5 miles/hr.) Cycling (11 miles/hr.) Badminton (competitive) Tennis (singles) Splitting wood Snow shoveling Hand lawn-mowing Folk (square) dancing Light downhill skiing Ski touring (2½ miles/hr.) Water skiing
8-10	Digging ditches Carrying 80 pounds Sawing hardwood	Jogging (5 miles/hr.) Cycling (12 miles/hr.) Horseback (gallop) Vigorous downhill skiing Basketball Mountain climbing Ice hockey Canoeing (5 miles/hr.) Touch football Paddleball
10-11	Shoveling at 10 lifts per minute (14-pound lifts)	Running (5½ miles/hr.) Cycling (13 miles/hr.) Ski touring in loose snow (4 miles/hr.) Squash racquets (social) Handball (social) Fencing Basketball (vigorous)

11+	Shoveling at 10 lifts per
	    minute (16-pound lifts)
		Running: 6 miles/hr.
		             7 miles/hr.
		             8 miles/hr.
		             9 miles/hr.
		           10 miles/hr.
		Ski touring in loose snow (5+ miles/hr.)
		Handball (competitive)
		Squash (competitive)

Your "Before" photo

Your "After" photo

Closing message

Congratulations! You've put together a year's worth of fitness, dedication to purpose, commitment. Hopefully you've given up the bathroom scale as a barometer of your fitness and have seen some redistribution of numbers in your body measurements. I sincerely trust that you've gradually changed over to eating more wholesome and nutritious foods, and that you've cut out some of the junk in your diet—and that you've established a stable eating pattern.

At this juncture, take a moment to look back at your past year. Take some time to page through your *Diary*. Your eyes will probably fall—at random—upon certain pages, and what you've written will call to mind some of the highlights of your year. Your notations will call to mind little moments here and there throughout the year. This is one of the wonderful things about paging through a diary, but especially through one that concentrates on how you are changing your life into something of which you can be especially proud.

Give yourself a pat on the back. You've come through brilliantly. You're on your way. Keep up the good work as you go into the next year. Your momentum is there; keep it on your side. Remember that you want to avoid inertia.

Go for it! And keep going for it all your life! It's worth it!

Elaine

Your fitness questionnaire

We would very much like to learn about your fitness. Why you found yourself gravitating toward a fitness lifestyle. How long you've been ''into'' fitness. What types of fitness activities you do. With this information, we will be better able to customize future editions of this *Diary*. We will also have a better idea of directions we can take to help you with your fitness in the future. When you've completed the questionnaire, please send it to me: Elaine LaLanne, The Jack LaLanne Company, P.O. Box 2, Hollywood, CA 90028. Please make sure to include your name and address; with that information, we will be better able to notify you of future fitness information that becomes available.

About You

Name _____

Street Address _____

City _____ State _____ Zip _____

Phone (optional) _____

1. Sex ☐ Male ☐ Female

2. Age ☐ 18 or below ☐ 19-25 ☐ 26-29 ☐ 30-35 ☐ 36-40 ☐ 41-45 ☐ 46-50 ☐ 51-55 ☐ 56-60 ☐ 60-65 ☐ 66-70 ☐ Older than 70

3. Height ☐ Below 4'8" ☐ 4'8"-4'10" ☐ 4'11"-5'0" ☐ 5'1"-5'3" ☐ 5'4"-5'6" ☐ 5'7"-5'9" ☐ 5'10"-6'0" ☐ 6'1"-6'3" ☐ 6'4" or above

4. Weight ☐ Below 80 lbs. ☐ 80-89 lbs. ☐ 90-99 lbs. ☐ 100-109 lbs. ☐ 110-119 lbs. ☐ 120-129 lbs. ☐ 130-139 lbs. ☐ 140-149 lbs. ☐ 150-159 lbs. ☐ 160-169 lbs. ☐ 170-179 lbs. ☐ 180-189 lbs. ☐ 190-199 lbs. ☐ 200-209 lbs. ☐ 210 lbs. or above

5. Marital status ☐ Married ☐ Single ☐ Divorced ☐ Widow/widower

6. Individual income ☐ Below $10,000 ☐ $10,000-19,999 ☐ $20,000-29,999 ☐ $30,000-39.999 ☐ $40,000-49,999 ☐ $50,000-59,999 ☐ $60,000-69,999 ☐ $70,000-79,999 ☐ $80,000-89,999 ☐ $90,000-99,999 ☐ $100,000 or above

7. Family income ☐ Below $10,000 ☐ $10,000-19,999 ☐ $20,000-29,999 ☐ $30,000-39,999 ☐ $40,000-49,999 ☐ $50,000-59,999 ☐ $60,000-69,999 ☐ $70,000-79,999 ☐ $80,000-89,999 ☐ $90,000-99,999 ☐ $100,000 or above

8. Education ☐ Did not graduate high school ☐ High school graduate ☐ Some college ☐ College graduate (2-year program) ☐ College graduate (4-year program) ☐ Some graduate school ☐ Master's degree ☐ Ph.D. or M.D.

9. Please fill in your current occupation (if retired, so indicate; if unemployed, indicate last full-time job; if housewife, indicate same). _____

10. How many members are there in your family? (By this, we mean how many people in total currently live with you in your residence; do not count children who have moved out and are on their own.) ☐ 1 (Myself) ☐ 2 ☐ 3 ☐ 4 ☐ 5 ☐ 6 ☐ 7 ☐ 8 ☐ 9 ☐ 10 or more

11. Do you have any pets? ☐ Dog(s) ☐ Cat(s) ☐ Horse(s) ☐ Gerbil(s)/Hamster(s) ☐ Bird(s) ☐ Other _____

12. Residence ☐ Own home ☐ Rent house ☐ Own condo ☐ Rent condo ☐ Rent apartment ☐ Live with family or friends ☐ Other _____

About Your Fitness

13. How long have you been involved in what you would consider a fitness lifestyle?
    ☐ I've just begun ☐ For 3-6 months ☐ For 6 months to a year ☐ 1-2 years ☐ 2-3 years
    ☐ 3-5 years ☐ 5-6 years ☐ 6-7 years ☐ 7-8 years ☐ 8-10 years ☐ 10 years or more.

14. How did you first get involved in fitness? ☐ I have always been involved in fitness
    ☐ Through a friend ☐ I looked at myself and resolved to do something to improve
    ☐ I wanted to improve my health ☐ I was looking for a challenge ☐ Other _____

15. What is your primary fitness activity? ☐ Proper diet ☐ General exercise ☐ Walking
    ☐ Running ☐ Bicycling ☐ Swimming ☐ Aerobic dance ☐ Jump rope ☐ Weight lifting
    ☐ Strength training ☐ Indoor exercising ☐ Going to a health spa ☐ Taking part in sports
    ☐ Other _____

16. How many days a week do you exercise? ☐ 1 ☐ 2 ☐ 3 ☐ 4 ☐ 5 ☐ 6 ☐ 7

17. Do you ever exercise more than once a day? ☐ Yes ☐ No

18. When you do engage in your exercise program, how long does it last? ☐ 5-15 minutes
    ☐ 15-30 minutes ☐ 30-45 minutes ☐ 45-60 minutes ☐ more than an hour ☐ It varies greatly
    Other _____

19. What is your resting pulse rate? _____ beats per minute

20. Have you ever been a cigarette smoker? ☐ Yes ☐ No

21. Do you currently smoke cigarettes? ☐ Yes ☐ No

22. Are you concerned about your diet and nutrition? ☐ Yes ☐ No

23. Are you currently involved in a diet of some sort? ☐ Yes ☐ No

24. If you are involved in a diet currently, which diet is it? _____

25. Do you believe that a diet alone is a route to fitness? ☐ Yes ☐ No ☐ Not certain

26. What is your primary source of fitness information? ☐ The daily newspaper ☐ News magazines
    ☐ Television information ☐ Magazines dealing with fitness ☐ My fitness instructor at the spa
    ☐ My doctor ☐ My fit friends ☐ I don't have a source, but would sure like to have one
    ☐ Other _____

27. What male and female do you most look up to as your ideal fit person?
    Male _____ Female _____

28. Do you ever find yourself trying to convince family and friends that they should adopt a fitness lifestyle?
    ☐ Yes ☐ No

29. What is the main reason you're involved in fitness? ☐ To look better ☐ To feel better
    ☐ To do something positive about my health ☐ To stop aging ☐ To keep my weight down
    ☐ To feel good about myself ☐ To make myself desirable for my mate
    ☐ To correct a health problem ☐ Because it is what's "in" today
    ☐ Because my friends are "into" it ☐ Because I'm concerned about the quality of my life
    ☐ To make up for how un-fit I was when I was younger ☐ Other _____

30. What type of information do you need about fitness?
    _____
    _____

31. How much money do you feel you spend per year on your fitness (including health spa
    memberships, clothing used for fitness, exercise equipment, etc.)?
    ☐ Less than $50 ☐ $50-100 ☐ $100-150 ☐ $150-250 ☐ $250-500 ☐ $500-750
    ☐ $750-1000 ☐ $1000-2000 ☐ $2000-5000 ☐ More than $5000

32. Please use the remaining space to tell me about your fitness:
    _____
    _____
    _____
    _____